Principles for the Selection of Doses in Chronic Rodent Bioassays

Principles for the Selection of Doses in Chronic Rodent Bioassays

Edited by Jeffery A. Foran

ILSI

International Life Sciences INSTITUTE

ILSI Risk Science Institute
Washington, D.C.

The **International Life Sciences Institute** (ILSI) is a nonprofit, worldwide foundation established in 1978 to advance the understanding of scientific issues relating to nutrition, food safety, toxicology, risk assessment, and the environment. ILSI also works to promote regulatory harmonization in these areas. By bringing together scientists from academia, government, industry, and the public sector, ILSI seeks a balanced approach to solving problems of common concern for the well-being of the general public. Headquartered in Washington, D.C., ILSI has branches in Argentina, Australia, Brazil, Europe, India, Japan, Korea, Mexico, North America, Southeast Asia, and Thailand, and a focal point in China.

Library of Congress Catalog Number: 97-71100

ILSI Press/ILSI Risk Science Institute
International Life Sciences Institute/Risk Science Institute
1126 Sixteenth Street, N. W.
Washington, D. C. 20036-4810

ISBN 0-944398-71-5
Printed in the United States of America

TABLE OF CONTENTS

Acknowledgments

This monograph is a distillation of 3 years of work by many people, most prominently the members of the ILSI Risk Science Institute working group on dose selection (members listed on page x). The entire working group is acknowledged as active contributors to this document. Drs. John Bucher, James Bus, Penny Fenner-Crisp, Jeffery Foran, Rogene Henderson, Steve Olin, James Swenberg, and Mike Watson served as members of a project steering committee, which was instrumental in the development of project goals and objectives. Andrea Gasper (ILSI Risk Science Institute) provided secretarial support throughout the project and Stephanie Carter (RSI) and Diane Dalisera (RSI) provided administrative support. Dr. Gino Scarano (RSI) provided valuable technical support during development of the monograph. The assistance of these individuals is acknowledged with thanks. Dr. Steve Olin, along with serving as a member of the steering committee and the working group, provided invaluable counsel and support throughout the project. The quality of this monograph would have been lessened considerably without his assistance.

This project was conducted under a cooperative agreement with the U.S. Environmental Protection Agency (EPA), Office of Pesticide Programs, Washington, D.C. Financial support was provided by the EPA and by the American Crop Protection Association. The financial support of these organizations is gratefully acknowledged.

Although the principles in Chapter 1 represent the consensus of the working group members, they do not necessarily represent the policies, positions, or opinions of their respective agencies and organizations. Additionally, material in Chapters 2 to 5, although contributed by members of the working group, also does not necessarily represent the policies, positions, or opinions of their respective agencies and organizations.

Members of the ILSI Risk Science Institute Working Group on Dose Selection

William T. Allaben
National Center for Toxicological Research
U.S. Food and Drug Administration
Jefferson, AR

John Ashby
Zeneca, Ltd.
Alderly Park
Cheshire, United Kingdom

Rolf Bass
European Agency for the Evaluation of Medicinal Products, United Kingdom
(formerly Federal Health Administration, Berlin, Germany)

John R. Bucher
National Toxicology Program
National Institute of Environmental Health Sciences
Research Triangle Park, NC

William Burnam
Office of Pesticide Programs
U.S. Environmental Protection Agency
Washington, DC

James S. Bus
Dow Chemical Company
Midland, MI

Byron E. Butterworth
Chemical Industry Institute of Toxicology
Research Triangle Park, NC

Michael Carakostas
The Coca-Cola Company
Atlanta, GA

Raymond A. Cardona
Uniroyal Chemical Company,
Bethany, CT

Samuel M. Cohen
University of Nebraska Medical Center
Omaha, NE

Joseph DeGeorge
Center for Drug Evaluation and Research
U.S. Food and Drug Administration
Rockville, MD

Bruce Domeyer
The Procter & Gamble Company
Cincinnati, OH

James Emerson
The Coca-Cola Company
Atlanta, GA

Penelope Fenner-Crisp
Office of Pesticide Programs
U.S. Environmental Protection Agency
Washington, DC

Jeffery A. Foran
ILSI Risk Science Institute
Washington, DC

David Gaylor
National Center for Toxicological Research
U.S. Food and Drug Administration
Jefferson, AR

Joyce F. Gee
Department of Pesticide Regulation
California Environmental Protection Agency
Sacramento, CA

Jay I. Goodman
Department of Pharmacology and Toxicology
Michigan State University
East Lansing, MI

Donald L. Grant
Pest Management Regulatory Agency
Health Canada
Ottawa, Ontario, Canada

David G. Hattan
Center for Food Safety and Applied Nutrition
U.S. Food and Drug Administration
Washington, DC

Yuzo Hayashi
Division of Risk Assessment
National Institute of Health Sciences
Tokyo, Japan

Rogene F. Henderson
Inhalation Toxicology Research Institute
Lovelace Biomedical and Environmental Research Institute
Albuquerque, NM

John L. Herrman
International Programme on Chemical Safety
World Health Organization
Geneva, Switzerland

Herman B. W. M. Koeter
Environment Directorate
Organization for Economic Cooperation and Development
Paris, France

Robert A. LeBoeuf
The Proctor & Gamble Company
Cincinnati, OH

Ronald J. Lorentzen
Office of Planning and Strategic Initiatives
U.S. Food and Drug Administration
Washington, DC

Ernest E. McConnell
Raleigh, NC

Kunitoshi Mitsumori
Department Of Pathology
Biological Safety Research Center
National Institute of Health Sciences
Tokyo, Japan

Stephen S. Olin
ILSI Risk Science Institute
Washington, DC

Jean Carol Parker
Office of Research and Development
U.S. Environmental Protection Agency
Washington, DC

Andrew Renwick
Clinical Pharmacology Group
University of Southampton
Southampton, UK

James T. Stevens
CIBA-GEIGY Ltd.
Basel, Switzerland

James A. Swenberg
Molecular Carcinogenesis and Mutagenesis
University of North Carolina
Chapel Hill, NC

Alan S. Taylor
BRI International
San Diego, CA (formerly U.S. Food and Drug Administration, Rockville, MD)

Marcia Van Gemert
Charles, Conn & Van Gemert
Charlotte Hall, MD (formerly U.S. Environmental Protection Agency)

Vanessa Vu
Office of Pollution Prevention and Toxics
U.S. Environmental Protection Agency
Washington, DC

Ronald Walker
School of Biological Sciences
University of Surrey
Guildford, Surrey, United Kingdom

Michael Watson
Pesticide Safety Directorate
Ministry of Agriculture, Fisheries, and Food
Hertfordshire, United Kingdom

K. Lemone Yielding
University of Texas Medical Branch
Galveston, TX

FOREWORD

One of the most debated issues in risk assessment has been the selection of doses for chronic animal bioassays. In 1984, the International Life Sciences Institute (Grice et al. 1984) identified 27 approaches or guidelines to dose selection for chronic animal bioassays that had been published between 1954 and 1980. Since 1980, dose selection has received no less attention and most recently has been the focus of efforts by the U.S. National Research Council (NRC) (1993), the European Centre for Ecotoxicology and Toxicology of Chemicals (1994), the International Federation of Societies of Toxicologic Pathologists (1992), and the International Conference on Harmonization of Technical Requirements for the Registration of Pharmaceuticals for Human Use (ICH2) (1995).

Perhaps the most contentious issue associated with dose selection is selection of the highest dose in carcinogenicity assays (McConnell 1989). In the 1960s, when chronic animal bioassays first were used routinely, the primary objective was to assess the qualitative potential for toxicity and carcinogenicity. For this purpose, the highest dose was selected to elicit a toxic but not life-threatening effect in a relatively small number of animals. However, with the advent of formal risk assessment methods in the late 1970s and early 1980s, studies that were originally intended to assess qualitatively the potential for toxicity or carcinogenicity were used to quantify adverse impacts; that is, to examine the shape and slope of the dose-response curve (Interagency Staff Group on Carcinogens [ISGC] 1986). Despite the change in interpretation and use of data from qualitative to both qualitative and quantitative purposes, criteria for dose selection (particularly the highest dose) remained remarkably constant (for example, compare Sontag et al. 1976 with ISGC principle 11 1986, Montesano et al. 1986, NRC 1993, and Haseman and Lockhart 1994). This consistency is even more remarkable in light of the advances that have occurred over the past 20 years in the understanding of mechanisms by which chemicals may induce cancer (Federal Register 1992).

A no less contentious problem in dose selection is the lack of international harmonization of selection procedures. Differences in dose-selection procedures that exist among many developed countries (discussed in Chapters 2 and 3) may lead to increased potential for trade barriers as a result of rejection of data from chronic bioassays designed to meet the requirements of one country and submitted for regulatory purposes in another. The ICH2 (1995) has reached agreement on procedures to select the highest dose in chronic bioassays for pharmaceuticals. However, no such consensus exists for pesticides, industrial chemicals, food additives, and other nonpharmaceutical chemicals.

The ILSI Risk Science Institute formed a working group in 1993 on dose selection for chronic animal bioassays as one of the activities under its cooperative agreement with the U.S. Environmental Protection Agency, Office of Pesticide Programs. In recognition of the dissatisfaction with current approaches to dose selection, the goal of the working group was to improve the testing of chemicals for long-term toxicity and carcinogenicity through appropriate dose selection and to work toward international harmonization of dose-selection procedures for chronic bioassays. The working group included scientists from academia, industry, and government representing the United States, Canada, Europe, and Japan.

This monograph, a product of the working group, contains sections that present a set of principles for dose selection in chronic rodent bioassays (Chapter 1); describe existing dose-selection requirements in various countries and agencies (Chapter 2); present case studies demonstrating the impact of international differences in dose-selection procedures (Chapter 3); examine factors that influence the selection of doses for chronic bioassays (Chapter 4); and present a series of case studies demonstrating how chemical-specific mechanistic considerations might influence dose selection (Chapter 5).

The principles presented in Chapter 1 represent the consensus of the Working Group on Dose Selection. There were divergent views among members of the working group regarding the nature and strength of the principles for dose selection. Some members felt that the principles were not strong enough, whereas others felt that they may be too prescriptive. However, all agreed that the principles for dose selection that are presented below are needed and are appropriate. Material in Chapters 2 to 5 contributed to and influenced the development of the principles that are presented in Chapter 1. The material in Chapters 2 to 5, however, represents the opinions of the individuals who contributed to those chapters.

Implementation of the principles presented in Chapter 1 will have two important benefits. First, implementation of the principles will improve the quality and consistency of the rodent bioassay, our most important tool to assess the long-term toxicity and carcinogenicity of chemicals, and lead to a better assessment of human risk. Second, international harmonization of dose-selection procedures will reduce the potential for trade barriers that may occur as a result of rejection of data designed to meet the requirements of one country and submitted for regulatory purposes in another.

REFERENCES

European Centre for Ecotoxicology and Toxicology of Chemicals (1994) Dose selection in chronic toxicity and carcinogenicity studies. Task force paper on MTD and limit doses. European Centre for Ecotoxicology and Toxicology of Chemicals, Brussels, Belgium

Federal Register (1992) NTP Board of Scientific Councilors Review of the NTP. Fed Register 57:31721–31730

Grice HC (ed) (1984) The selection of doses in chronic toxicity/carcinogenicity studies. Springer Verlag, New York, pp 9–49

Haseman JK, Lockhart A (1994) The relationship between the use of the maximum tolerated dose and study sensitivity for detecting rodent carcinogenicity. Fund Appl Toxicol 22:382–394

Interagency Staff Group on Carcinogens (ISGC), US (1986) Chemical carcinogens: A review of the science and its associated principles. Environ Health Perspec 67:201–282

International Conference on Harmonization of Technical Requirements for Registration of Pharmaceuticals for Human Use (ICH2) (1995) Fed Register 60:11278 (March 1995)

International Federation of Societies of Toxicologic Pathologists (1992) IFSTP guidelines for the design and interpretation of the chronic rodent carcinogenicity bioassay. Exp Toxicol Pathol 44:443–456

McConnell EE (1989) The maximum tolerated dose: The debate. J Am College Toxicol 8:115–120

Montesano R, Bartsch H, Vainio H, et al (1986) Long-term and short-term assays for carcinogens: A critical appraisal. IARC Scientific Publication 83. International Agency for Research on Cancer, Lyons, France

National Research Council (1993) Issues in Risk Assessment. National Academy Press, Washington, DC

Sontag JM, Page NP, Saffiotti U (1976) Guidelines for carcinogen bioassay in small rodents. National Institutes of Health, DHEW Publication No. (NIH) 76-801. National Institutes of Health, Bethesda, MD

Chapter 1

Principles for Dose Selection in Chronic Rodent Bioassays

INTRODUCTION

The selection of doses for chronic rodent bioassays requires many scientific judgments, based in part on toxicologic information (from prechronic studies and other sources), potential exposure, chemical structure and activity, chemical use, and others. All of the principles presented in this chapter may not be pertinent for every chemical; however, many factors and endpoints are identified that should be utilized to guide dose selection for chronic bioassays.

The principles presented in this chapter and in the monograph as a whole do not provide a "cookbook" for dose selection, nor do they provide detailed instructions for their use. Rather, this chapter provides general principles that incorporate sound science and concurrently encourage efforts to select the highest dose that maximizes study sensitivity while producing results that are biologically and toxicologically credible. The results of cancer bioassays are often the basis for cancer risk assessments of environmental chemicals; therefore, the incorporation of sound scientific principles in selection of middle and lower doses for chronic bioassays is also encouraged.

Doses selected for chronic studies may depend on or be influenced by strain, species, route of administration, mode of administration, diet, and other factors. There are also critically important issues associated with interpretation of the results of chronic bioassays in the context of risk assessment.[1] Despite the importance of these issues, this chapter presents principles that focus, like the remainder of the monograph, solely on dose selection for chronic rodent bioassays. Further, although the focus of the monograph is on dose selection for bioassays of environmental chemicals, some of the factors that influence dose selection for pharmaceuticals are relevant for environmental chemicals; thus, these factors were considered during the working group's

---

[1]Discussion of dose selection occurs throughout this monograph in the context of quantitative risk assessment and the specific steps of that process (e.g., hazard identification, dose-response assessment). The working group was aware of the Joint OECD/IPCS project on Harmonization of Terminology used in Risk Assessment; therefore, no effort was made to reach consensus on the definition of terms.

deliberations and during development of the principles presented below. However, the following recommendations for dose selection of environmental chemicals are not necessarily intended to address, nor do they necessarily apply to, studies of pharmaceutical compounds.

PRINCIPLES

Principle 1

Dose selection for chronic studies must be based on sound toxicologic principles. Within a reasonable dose range, increasing the dose can increase the ability to detect an effect; therefore, doses for chronic rodent bioassays should be selected within this range to maximize the sensitivity of a chronic bioassay. However, trying to increase study sensitivity by increasing doses into ranges that do not reflect application of sound toxicologic principles could lead to results that are inappropriate for human risk assessment.

Increasing the highest dose in a chronic bioassay may increase sensitivity within some defined dose range, but the potential exists that different mechanisms of toxicity or chemical mode of action are active at higher doses, which may not be relevant to humans exposed to lower doses. In this case, selection of the highest dose may be influenced by consideration of the mechanism/mode of action and other factors discussed in Principle 4. However, when the highest dose in a carcinogenicity assay is limited by effects (e.g., a mode of action in one organ system) that are thought not to occur in humans, one must be aware that it still is possible that a higher dose of the chemical may be carcinogenic in other animal/organ systems.

To address these issues, the working group encourages an approach to dose selection that incorporates all relevant information from prechronic studies and other sources, uses toxicologic tools associated with an understanding of the mechanisms or mode of action by which a chemical produces an effect (e.g., genotoxicity, cell proliferation, etc.), and uses good scientific principles to enhance the accuracy of judgments of potential human risks. In the case of negative studies (particularly where the highest dose is chosen based on a full characterization of the chemical's toxicity in prechronic studies), use of sound scientific principles as well as all available chemical, physical, and toxicologic data will lessen concern that the result may be a false negative. Similarly, in positive carcinogenicity studies, this approach will lessen concern that the result may be a false positive. In both cases, the predictiveness of the bioassay for human health effects will be improved.

Principle 2

A chronic bioassay requires a major investment in resources and time, and the objective of such a study should be broader than hazard identification. Scientists who conduct chronic bioassays and those who use data from bioassays, including regulatory agencies, should encourage innovative approaches to dose selection by considering appropriate study designs, mechanistic data, and other information in the design and interpretation of studies. Use of additional endpoints and other information must be based on sound scientific rationale, and such designs should be evaluated on the basis of their individual merits.

A goal of high-dose selection in carcinogenicity bioassays is, in the context of hazard identification, to reduce the likelihood of a false-negative result. However, it is recognized that the qualitative nature of the hazard (e.g., carcinogenic response) may itself be dose dependent. This principle encourages approaches to dose selection that incorporate consideration of mechanistic and other toxicologic information. Such approaches should improve the scientific basis for dose selection and aid in interpretation of data generated from chronic bioassays.

Principle 3

Human exposure should be considered in dose selection, particularly for selection of the middle and lowest doses. Further, the middle and lowest doses should be selected to characterize the shape of the dose-response curve as much as possible. Selection of the middle and lower doses should take into account factors such as the mechanism or mode of action, toxicokinetics, and others listed in Principles 4 and 5 and should not be based solely on a fraction of the highest dose.

Issues that should be considered when incorporating potential human exposure in dose selection include the human exposure route and mode, the dose range in the chronic bioassay in relation to human exposure, and the duration and frequency of human exposure, if known. Subpopulations that may be more highly exposed than the general population, or that are genetically more susceptible, also should be considered. The relationship between external and delivered (internal) dose (e.g., ingested dose versus dose delivered to the target organ, pharmacokinetics) in both humans and test organisms may influence dose selection. Further, for substances expected to exhibit a toxicity threshold, or if the evaluation of carcinogenic potential is being combined with an evaluation of chronic toxicity, the study should be designed to include one dose that does not elicit adverse effects; that is, one dose should be a NOAEL. Of course, caution must be exercised to ensure that the NOAEL is not simply an artifact of small sample size or poor study design.

Principle 4

The working group has recommended the use of innovative approaches, additional endpoints, and other information in the selection of doses for chronic rodent bioassays. The following endpoints, generally determined in prechronic studies, should be considered in dose selection for chronic rodent bioassays. Further, it is recognized that endpoints other than those listed below may provide important information for dose selection, and use of those endpoints, where they are based on sound toxicologic principles, is encouraged. Such endpoints may be available presently, or they may be developed as the science of toxicology advances.

Histopathology

The site, morphology, and severity of the treatment-related effects observed in the prechronic study must be taken into account in setting dose levels for the chronic study. Histopathologic examination of tissues, especially the liver, gastrointestinal tract, urinary tract, respiratory tract, skin, spleen/bone marrow/blood, and endocrine tissues derived from properly designed prechronic studies, often provides information that is crucial for dose selection in chronic bioassays.

Toxicokinetics

Studies to determine the effect of dose (or exposure concentration) on absorption, tissue distribution, metabolism, and clearance of a compound are helpful in selecting appropriate doses for the chronic bioassay. The kinetics of absorption will determine the internal dose achieved. The absorption and clearance of the compound and its metabolites will determine the systemic and target organ exposure resulting from a single dose and can be used to design the treatment regimen required to achieve a desired internal dose. The effect of repeated exposures on the pattern of absorption, metabolism, detoxification, and clearance of a compound will provide information on the internal dose achieved during chronic exposure under conditions of the bioassay.

Cell Proliferation

In the process of chemical carcinogenesis, events related to induced cell proliferation may be critical in fixing mutations and in providing a selective growth advantage to precancerous cells. Considerations may be different for direct mitogenic stimulation of organ growth versus regenerative cell proliferation, and these modes of action should be distinguished for the test agent. Further, apoptosis can be a strong determinant of normal and precancerous cell turnover kinetics and should be considered. Information on the dose dependence of regenerative cell proliferation is a useful adjunct to histologic observations in determining the shapes of organ-specific toxic response curves. This information can be of value in selecting high, middle, and low doses and in interpreting the results of the study.

Physiologic Function

Disturbances of physiology or homeostasis that would compromise the validity of the study should be considered in the dose-selection process. Examples include hypotension, inhibition of blood clotting, overwhelming normal pulmonary clearance mechanisms, immune system effects, and in some cases hormonal imbalance. Such disturbances, and their effects on the validity of a study, may be difficult to determine and may apply differentially to different categories of chemicals (e.g., pharmaceuticals in which the desired pharmacologic action is a physiologic effect).

Body Weight

It is suggested that if body-weight changes are the primary factor in the selection of the highest-dose group (that is, when no other toxic effects are observed), a decrement in body-weight gain of no more than 5–10% in prechronic studies should be used in the selection of the highest dose for chronic assays of carcinogenicity.

Historically, scientists have adopted a 10% decreased body-weight gain at the end of prechronic studies (typically 90 days duration) as the target that should not be exceeded in chronic (carcinogenicity) studies. It is now recognized that there is a positive correlation between body weight and the occurrence of certain tumors in rodent species and strains used in safety assessment or for hazard identification; i.e., the higher the body weight between 6 and 18 months on test, the higher the probability that the animal will develop some tumors. Moreover, the lower the body weight, the less sensitive the animal may be to agent-induced toxicity, including cancer. A substantial decrease in body-weight gain therefore could reduce the animal's ability to respond to compound-induced toxicities.

Clinical Chemistry, Hematology, Urinalysis

Clinical chemistry and urinalysis results are best used to support dose-selection decisions based on other criteria/parameters. Changes in serum clinical chemistry in the absence of histopathologic observations may not affect high-dose selection but may complement dose-selection decisions based on toxicokinetics, cell proliferation, and other parameters. Hematology results also are more often affected secondarily to other processes more relevant for dose selection (e.g., inflammation). However, when hematologic tissues are determined to be a target organ in prechronic studies, hematology results may be an appropriate basis for dose selection.

Organ Weights

Organ weights are not often the critical factor in selection of doses for chronic rodent bioassays. Chemically induced changes in organ weights, however, should be considered in conjunction with other data in the dose-selection process.

Ideally, data from the factors and endpoints listed above would be collected from prechronic studies and used to select doses for chronic studies; however, not all parameters may be useful or necessary for every compound. Even when based on information concerning the points described above, dose selection for a chronic bioassay will remain an inexact process; thus, reconsideration of these same points must be made when interpreting and assessing the significance of the effects obtained in the bioassay.

Principle 5

Physicochemical factors (e.g., solubility, vapor pressure), the bioavailability of the compound, the palatability of the compound in food or drinking water, and other factors such as the potential for the substance to cause adverse effects at the site of administration (e.g., irritation, erosion, and ulceration) will influence the selection of the highest dose for chronic rodent bioassays. It is recommended that doses for chronic rodent bioassays be selected to minimize or avoid adverse nutritional, physical, organoleptic, and irritant effects.

When given in the diet, the general default upper dose has been limited to a range of 2–5% by weight in the diet of the test animal, unless the substance is likely to occur in large amounts in the human diet (i.e., is a macronutrient). For gavage dosing, the daily dose is commonly limited to 1–2 g per kg of body weight. Country- and agency-specific applications of this principle are discussed in greater detail in Chapter 2.

CONCLUSIONS

The ILSI Risk Science Institute working group on dose selection strongly encourages the generation of data through use of the principles presented in this chapter in selecting the highest, middle, and lowest doses for chronic bioassays. Concurrently, the working group encourages a move away from sole reliance on body weight and histopathology as the primary criteria for high-dose selection in chronic rodent bioassays. At the completion of the bioassay, one should look retrospectively at the doses that were selected and at the data generated at those doses. Data obtained from doses that are inconsistent with the principles presented in this chapter may not be appropriate for use in human health risk assessment. Use of sound scientific principles as well as all available chemical, physical, and toxicologic data, particularly those presented in the principles in this chapter, will improve the process of identifying and selecting doses for chronic bioassays and is recommended by the working group.

Chapter 2

National and International Dose Selection Requirements[1]

OVERVIEW

Achieving the international harmonization of dose selection procedures requires insight into similarities and differences among existing country and organization guidelines. To that end, dose-selection procedures, the regulatory basis for those procedures, and the intended use of data derived from studies that utilize those procedures in Europe, Japan, Canada, and the United States are presented and examined in this chapter. Also examined are the guidelines developed by the International Conference on Harmonization (ICH-2) and the Organization for Economic Cooperation and Development (OECD). Wherever possible, dose-selection procedures were examined for pesticides and industrial chemicals, pharmaceuticals, and food additives.

Virtually every country/organization requires a highest dose in chronic rodent (carcinogenicity) bioassays that does not induce overt toxicity and is not predicted to shorten the lifespan of test animals except as a result of neoplastic development (language taken from guidelines of the European Union). Despite the widespread use of the concept of no overt toxicity to select the highest dose, there is a perception that both terminology and the precise definition of the highest dose differ dramatically among countries and organizations. This perception has been reinforced by an examination conducted by the International Life Sciences Institute (Grice et al. 1984), which identified 27 different approaches or guidelines to dose selection for chronic animal bioassays that had been published between 1954 and 1980 (Table 1).

Despite the perception of significant international differences in dose-selection procedures, there is, nonetheless, a great deal of similarity between dose-selection procedures both in the terminology and in the guidance provided to select doses. For example, most countries/organizations specify the highest dose as the maximum tolerated dose (MTD; United States, Japan, Canada, OECD, ICH-2), although some countries/organizations use terms such as minimally toxic dose (European Union) or maximum feasible dose (MFD;

---

[1]Contributions to this chapter were made by R. Bass, J. R. Bucher, R. S. Chhabra, J. DeGeorge, M. R. Elwell, P. Fenner-Crisp, J. F. Gee, D. L. Grant, D. G. Hattan, Y. Hayashi, H. B.W. M. Koeter, K. Mitsumori, A. S. Taylor, V. Vu, and M. Watson.

Table 1. Methods for high-dose selection for chronic rodent bioassays (from Grice et al. 1984)

Reference	High-dose selection guidelines
Barnes and Denz 1954	Produces some toxic reactions. On a body-weight basis, up to 100× greater than the estimated daily intake by humans. Fitzhugh 1955, Weisburger and Weisburger, 1967, Benitz,
1970, D'Aguanno 1974, Dept. of Health and Social Security (UK) 1979	Level that approaches the tolerated amount and produces a "menacing" effect on the animals as a whole or on one or more vital organs.
Clayson 1962	The test substance should be presented to the target tissue in as high a concentration as possible without killing or seriously weakening the test animal.
Della Porta 1964, Loomis 1968 (carc.), Berenblum 1969, WHO 1969, Magee 1970	Should induce some toxic effect, but treatment should be stopped in time to avoid loss of too many animals.
Loomis 1968 (chronic)	Toxicologic signs are necessary, but if toxicity progresses toward lethality, the group is divided into two subgroups, one of which no longer receives the test substance.
FDA panel 1971	Doses chosen so that they result in experimental conditions likely to yield maximum tumor incidence. Dose that is several orders of magnitude above actual use level.
Peck 1974, Newberne 1975	Largest amount tolerated without observable toxic effects, including depressed growth rate or decreased food intake, as determined in studies of 3 to 12 months duration (drug studies).
Friedman 1974	(1) Will not produce weight depression of >10% vs. Controls (rodents) or weight difference of 10% between control and treated animals of other species. (2) Allows for at least 50% of treated animals to survive to the end of the study, provided that intercurrent infections do not reduce viability of the test animals. (3) Will not produce pharmacologic effects that will interfere with completion of the study or otherwise invalidate the result.

Japan, Canada, United States, ICH-2). These terms are not necessarily mutually exclusive. Specific guidance for selection of the highest dose (MTD, minimally toxic dose, MFD, etc.) in chronic rodent bioassays also is provided by most countries/organizations (Table 2).

Most countries/organizations consider decreases in body-weight gain (as elicited in prechronic studies) as an important determinant of the highest dose.

Table 1. Methods for high-dose selection for chronic rodent bioassays (from Grice et al. 1984) (continued)

Reference	High-dose selection guidelines
Health and Welfare Canada 1975	Should not markedly shorten the life span of the animals compared to controls but should be sufficiently high to produce slight but noticeable effects on weight gain, food consumption, or some other relevant physiological parameter.
Sontag et al 1976, Page 1977a, 1977b, Interagency Regulatory Liaison Group 1979	MTD should not alter the animals' longevity from effects other than carcinogenicity; causes no more than a 10% weight decrement compared to appropriate control group; does not produce mortality, clinical signs of toxicity, or pathologic lesions (other than those that may be related to neoplastic response) that would be predicted to shorten the animals' natural life span.
Food Safety Council 1978, CEC 1980, IARC 1980	That dose in a subchronic (90 day) study that: (1) induces no overt toxicity, i.e., appreciable death of cells or organ dysfunction as determined by appropriate clinical pathological or biochemical methods; (2) induces no toxic manifestations that are predicted to shorten the life span of the animals except as the result of neoplastic development; (3) does not retard weight gain during the subchronic test by >10% as compared to control animals; (4) takes into consideration metabolic and pharmacokinetic data, and, if dose-dependent qualitative or quantitative differences occur, at least one test dose should be set above the metabolic shift.
WHO 1978	Should produce some slight evidence of toxicity but be compatible with normal physiological function.
OECD 1981	Elicit some signs of toxicity without causing excessive lethality (chronic toxicity tests) or without substantially altering normal life span due to effects other than tumors (cancer tests). Signs of toxicity are those that may be indicated by alterations in serum enzyme levels or slight depression of body-weight gain (<10%). For diet mixture, the ingested concentration should not exceed 5%.

However, there does not appear to be exclusive reliance on this endpoint to define the highest dose in any country/organization. Rather, other endpoints, including information on metabolic saturation, histopathology, and toxicokinetics, are used to guide selection of the highest dose (Table 2), although the degree of reliance on one or a set of endpoints is not clearly defined in country/organization-specific guidance.

Although there is considerable similarity in dose-selection procedures among countries and organizations, complete concordance in the guidance for selection of the highest and lower doses does not exist. Further, many entities

Table 2. Considerations in dose selection for chronic rodent bioassays

Chemical class	Country/ organization	Considerations in high dose selection	Considerations in selection of lower doses
Pharmaceuticals	All	Pharmacodynamic endpoints, toxicity-based endpoints (MTD), pharmacokinetic endpoints, saturation of absorption, MFD.	Two doses between control and high dose. Consider toxicokinetics, metabolic pathways, human exposure, response in rodents, rodent physiology, mechanistic information.
Pesticides and industrial chemicals	EPA	Mortality; body-weight gain; clinical signs—hematology, clinical chemistry, organ weights, organ morphology, histopathology.	Two doses in addition to control and high dose. Lowest dose should produce no biologically significant toxicity. Middle dose should be set between high and low dose.
	European Union	Depression in body-weight gain, tissue necrosis, metabolic saturation, minimal target organ toxicity.	Provide information to assess relevance to humans, human exposure, pharmacodynamic and toxicity data, rodent physiology, mechanistic information.
	Japan	Body-weight gain; mortality. No more than 5% of diet.	Not applicable
	Canada	Body-weight gain, clinical signs, diet consumed, hematology, urinalysis, clinical chemistry, pathology, histology, metabolism, toxicokinetics.	Two doses in addition to high dose and control. Lowest dose should produce no toxicity. Doses should be sufficiently different to elicit distinct responses.

Table 2. Considerations in dose selection for chronic rodent bioassays (continued)

Chemical class	Country/ organization	Considerations in high dose selection	Considerations in selection of lower doses
Pesticides and industrial chemicals	NTP	Mortality, body-weight gain, target organ histopathology, toxicokinetic information, cell proliferation.	Two doses between high dose and controls. Fractions of high dose. Other considerations including toxicokinetics, cell proliferation, etc.
	OECD	Minimal toxicity, body-weight gain, serum enzyme levels.	Interference with normal growth and development, low dose not lower than 10% of high dose. Also consider toxicokinetic properties.
Food additives	FDA	Mortality; body-weight gain; organ weight changes; histopathological modifications; alterations in hematologic, urinary, and clinical chemistry parameters.	Two dose groups in addition to high dose and control. Lowest dose should not elicit toxicity or be lower than 10% of high dose.
	European Union	Nutritional imbalance, metabolic overload, physiology and biochemistry, body-weight gain, metabolic and pharmacokinetic/ toxicokinetic information. No more than 5% of diet.	Not applicable
	Japan	Body-weight gain, mortality, MFD (5% of diet).	Not applicable
	Canada	Body-weight gain,. clinical signs, diet consumed, hematology, urinalysis, clinical chemistry, pathology, histology, metabolism, toxicokinetics.	Two doses in addition to high dose and control. Lowest dose should produce no toxicity. Doses should be sufficiently different to elicit distinct responses.

indicate that specific guidance for dose selection will not be provided; rather, doses for chronic rodent bioassays should be selected on a case-by-case basis. Therefore, international differences in dose-selection procedures do exist, particularly where a country/organization relies more or less heavily than other entities on one or a few endpoints (e.g., decreases in body-weight gain). In the following sections of this chapter, country- and organization-specific guidance for dose-selection procedures as well as for use and interpretation of data derived from chronic rodent bioassays is provided. In Chapter 3, the implications of these differences for international trade are examined through a series of chemical-specific case studies.

EUROPE

Background

Until recently, regulatory control of pesticides and industrial chemicals in Europe has not been coordinated at anything other than the national level. Within the European Union, testing requirements for industrial chemicals are now defined by the latest revisions of a directive adopted by the Council of the European Union relating to the classification, packaging, and labeling of dangerous substances. The so-called dangerous substances directive, adopted in 1967 (67/548/EEC [European Economic Community]), has been amended seven times; the seventh amendment was adopted in 1992 (92/32/EEC). The dangerous substances directive details the annual and cumulative production figures that need to be attained before further data are generated.

The European Union has recently adopted a registration directive for pesticides (91/414/EEC). Compared to the dangerous substances directive, authorization of specific uses of pesticides results in considerably more data being generated on fewer chemicals. This is because authorization for use of a pesticide requires a broad range of data to be generated and evaluated before it can be introduced onto the market, whereas fewer data need to be generated before introduction of an industrial chemical into commerce.

Whether carcinogenicity data are generated for pesticides or industrial chemicals, the same general principles of study design and dose selection apply. Both sets of legislation make specific reference to EEC test methods, although studies conducted in accordance with OECD protocols also would be acceptable. When required, long-term carcinogenicity studies are generally carried out in two species—the rat and the mouse. Tests in other species are rarely reported.

Chronic bioassay data for pesticides and industrial chemicals are generally evaluated in the same manner. The first step is to provide a qualitative evaluation of the potential of a chemical to cause a carcinogenic response in the test species. Tumor incidence in treated animals initially is compared with the incidence in untreated, concurrent controls. Information on induction time is available only for tumors that cause death or that have clinically visible signs. These data, if available, also will be taken into account, as will background knowledge of tumor incidence in the test species and strain, so that a low incidence of an unusual tumor type is not ignored. Historical control data often are used in this evaluation, but these data must be relevant. Consideration of species, strain, animal supplier, location, and duration of the study are all examples of factors to be considered in deciding the relevance of historical control data. If there is no indication of carcinogenicity in the test species in a well-conducted study, this information also contributes to the regulatory decision-making process.

If evidence of carcinogenicity is found, the next step is to examine all the available data to try to determine the mechanistic basis of the response in the test species. As far as pesticides are concerned, if the carcinogenicity is directly associated with genotoxicity considered relevant to humans, then it is highly unlikely that any approval for use that leaves residues in food would be granted.

In the case of nongenotoxic carcinogens, to determine the relevance of the effect observed in the test species to potential effects in humans, mechanistic data are considered on a case-by-case basis. From the available scientific evidence in some cases, the regulatory process may conclude that the effect seen in the test animal would not occur at all in humans and therefore can be ignored for purposes of extrapolation to humans. In other cases, it may be concluded that the carcinogenic effect in the test animals is associated with a phenomenon that exhibits a nonlinear dose-response relationship, so that a no-observed-adverse-effect level (NOAEL) can be established for at least one element of the underlying mode of action, which has led to the carcinogenic effect. In these cases, it is possible that a margin of exposure/safety may be used based on the NOAEL for the underlying mode of action, and a regulatory decision can be made by comparing the NOAEL with predicted human exposure.

European authorities, when evaluating data from chronic bioassays, tend to approach each evaluation as a separate scientific exercise. Currently, there are no formal written guidelines for assessment procedures.

The acceptability of studies, once reports are provided to the relevant authority, is generally decided on a case-by-case basis, using scientific judgment. There are no defined evaluation procedures that differentiate an acceptable study from one that is rejected. Although this can lead to differences in decision making between different regulatory authorities in some instances, such cases are rare, because the regulatory approach is to use the data that have been supplied to make a decision. Uncertainties in the data are reflected by the use of increased uncertainty (or safety) factors used in derivation of reference doses or by rejection of the entire application for approval rather than by formal rejection of a specific study.

The Commission of the European Communities (CEC 1989), in its advice on the presentation of a food-additive petition, states that "no fixed programme is laid down to be followed in every case" and refers to World Health Organization (WHO) and OECD protocols for those undertaking toxicity studies. Insight into the view of European regulators can be obtained from the reports of the Scientific Committee for Food (CEC 1990), which recommends that "combined protocols are used for studying chronic toxicity and carcinogenicity in the same experiment."

In the United Kingdom, guidelines for the design of animal safety testing have been developed by the Committee on Toxicity (CoT) and by the Committee on Carcinogenicity (CoC 1991). The CoT guidelines (CoT 1982) in relation to subacute tests state that:

> for essentially non-toxic substances (e.g., potential major food constituents) it may not be possible to test at dose levels substantially above the human exposure range without distorting the animals' diet to the point at which 'toxic effects' occur non-specifically for this reason.

In the European Union, chronic bioassays usually are required for pharmaceutical development when the drug will be used continuously for 6 months or longer (requirements for shorter and intermittent use are less clearly defined and less foreseeable) or when the biological, biotechnological, chemical, or pharmacodynamic class of the compound to be investigated has raised suspicion because of its structure, activity, or toxicity (including genotoxicity, short-term testing for carcinogenicity, and chronic administration). A risk-benefit assessment, evaluation, and decision will be made that takes into account the uniqueness of the therapeutic activity, available therapeutic alternatives, and the situation of the patient. For example, strong alkylating agents have been marketed for treatment of serious, life-threatening conditions such as cancer; weak carcinogens have not been approved when the indication is less serious or other medicines are available. Such an assessment generally is performed for the whole population "at risk" rather than for a "single patient."

Dose Selection

Pesticides and Industrial Chemicals

Early consultation with regulatory authorities to discuss study design and dose-level selection is not common in the European Union. The regulatory process, particularly for pesticides, is designed to assess applications for approval of specified uses and has no facility to allow for "approval" of study designs or dose levels. Dose levels used in studies are based on the results of preliminary, shorter-term studies; again, reference is made to EEC test methods or OECD protocols. Although the term MTD has been used in reference to selection of the highest dose tested, in contrast to the concept in the United States of MTD, the European interpretation is sometimes better defined as a minimally toxic dose as follows (European Communities—91/414/EEC 1991 and subsequently updated with the following directives: 93/71/EEC, 94/37/EEC, 94/79/EEC, 95/35/EEC, and 95/36/EEC):

> The doses tested, including the highest dose tested, must be selected on the basis of the results of short-term testing and where available at the time of planning the studies concerned, on the basis of metabolism and toxicokinetic data. The highest dose level in carcinogenicity studies should elicit signs of minimal toxicity such as slight depression in body weight gain (less than 10%), without causing tissue necrosis or metabolic saturation and without substantially altering normal life span due to effects other than tumors. If the long-term toxicity study is carried out separately, the highest dose level should elicit definite signs of toxicity without causing excessive lethality. Higher doses, causing excessive toxicity are not considered relevant to evaluations to be made.

Regardless of the method used for selection of the highest dose, the selection of the middle and lowest doses for the carcinogenicity study should provide information to aid in assessing the relevance of study findings to humans. The doses should be selected after integration of rodent and human exposure with pharmacodynamic and toxicity data. The rationale for the selection of these doses should be provided. Although not all-encompassing, the following points should be considered in selection of the middle and lowest doses for rodent carcinogenicity studies: 1) linearity of toxicokinetics and saturation of metabolic pathways, 2) human exposure, 3) pharmacodynamic response in rodents, 4) alterations in normal rodent physiology, 5) mechanistic information and potential for threshold effects, and 6) the unpredictability of the progression of toxicity observed in short-term studies.

Food Additives

Food additives, by their nature and functionality, normally show very low acute and subchronic toxicity. In consequence, the selection of doses for chronic toxicity and carcinogenicity studies often is limited by the tolerance of the animal to diet manipulation and the potential for producing irrelevant effects because of nutritional imbalances, metabolic overload, and abnormal physiology and biochemistry unrelated to a direct action of the test compound.

The Scientific Committee for Food (CEC 1990) uses the same phrase as the CEC (i.e., "most of the procedures for carrying out such studies are relatively standardized but several areas are still considered controversial") but then addresses a number of issues including dose selection, in relation to which the report states:

> It is suggested that three dose levels apart from controls should be tested. The highest level chosen should be the one which in subchronic tests induces no overt toxicity or toxic manifestations, and is predicted not to shorten the life- span of the animals except as a result of neoplastic development. Furthermore, it should not retard the weight gain by more than 10% as compared to control animals, and should take into account metabolic and pharmacokinetic data.

It is clear from this description that the top dose could approach a MTD but that it should not exceed the MTD; in other words, the MTD is a cutoff rather than a target for the top dose.

The problem of producing nutritional artifacts also is recognized as the report further states:

> For food additives, which are essentially non-toxic chemicals, it may prove impossible to identify a dose level which is toxic, or the administration at the maximum tolerated level may entail such major alterations to the composition of the diet that a meaningful experiment is impossible. The administration of doses of any compound at dose levels in excess of 5% of the diet may cause non-specific chronic toxic effects and these may in turn influence tumor incidence non-specifically. In such cases the highest dose level should generally be set at 5% of the diet.

Dose selection for chronic toxicity and carcinogenicity was considered in the CoC guidelines (CoC 1991), which contain some important insights:

> The general aim is to maximize exposure, tempered by toxicokinetic and toxicity considerations; but it is equally important, especially on oral tests on inactive substances or macro-ingredients of the diet, not to disturb the normal nutrition and health of the animals by giving too large a dose or by making the diet unpalatable.

It is recommended that the highest dose in a study should usually be set at the MTD, and there is a detailed interpretation by the CoC of what is meant by MTD:

> The maximum tolerated dose is selected first by reference to the toxicokinetics of the compound (or a marker component of a mixture); it should in general be as high as possible provided that other undesirable effects are not found (e.g., saturation of normal absorption or metabolic

pathways). Next, evidence about the toxic effects of that dose level over a period of several weeks to few months should be reviewed. A dose producing continuing necrosis or other severe tissue damage needs to be avoided because it will jeopardize survival and compromise interpretation of the results. If the substance does not cause specific target organ toxicity or a gross functional effect, the high dose level is conventionally set as a dose likely to cause about 10% reduction in weight gain over the life span of the animals to be used; it is commonly chosen from the results of a preliminary 90-day toxicity test and multi-dose kinetic studies. A further constraint is that the top dose of a substance should not normally exceed 5% of the weight of the diet or drinking water. The reasons for selecting particular doses should be clearly stated in the final report, including such relevant toxicokinetic data as blood levels, areas under the curve and metabolic pattern.

This description indicates that the MTD is a target level rather than either a minimum level to ensure acceptable assay sensitivity or a maximum level or cutoff above which results would be of doubtful relevance to human safety evaluation.

Pharmaceuticals

The regulation of pharmaceuticals in the European Union currently follows the ICH guidelines for dose selection, which are presented in detail later in this chapter.

JAPAN

Background

During the past 2 decades, five carcinogenicity test guidelines or guidances have been issued by the responsible ministry or agency of the Japanese government for pharmaceuticals (Ministry of Health and Welfare [MHW] 1984), environmental chemicals (MHW 1990), agricultural chemicals (Ministry of Agriculture, Forestry and Fisheries [MAFF] 1985), veterinary drugs (MHW 1988), and feed additives (MHW 1989).

The toxicity of chemicals to humans is currently evaluated on the basis of analyzing/integrating data derived from a series of studies including various toxicity tests, toxicokinetic/metabolic studies, and mechanistic studies. During this evaluation process, results of chronic toxicity bioassays have been used in Japan for two major purposes in elucidating toxicologic properties of test chemicals.

The first purpose is to assess whether long-term administration of the test chemical might be associated with any morphologic lesions or functional disturbances that would not be evident in animals receiving only short-term administration. Data on the occurrence of neoplastic or degenerative lesions as well as acceleration of age-related organ changes can be raised as pieces of information necessary for this purpose.

The second purpose is to clarify the toxicologic or medical implications of short-term bioassay findings for two issues. The first issue concerns quantitative or semiquantitative comparison of the dose-response data between short-term bioassays and chronic bioassays. For example, it is clearly necessary with respect to safety evaluation to determine whether long-term administration of the chemical at the MTD determined in short-term studies can cause any adverse effects in animals. The second issue is to correlate target effects of the test chemical between short-term and chronic bioassays. For example, we must be able to judge whether the occurrence of pulmonary fibrosis in chronic bioassays can be regarded as a sequel to long-term sustained pneumotoxicity of a test chemical causing alveolar damage in a short-term bioassay. Evaluation of nongenotoxic carcinogens also represents a pertinent example of this issue.

Unlike the case with genotoxic carcinogens, general criteria for nongenotoxic carcinogens have not yet been established, because many different examples of effects exerted through a variety of mechanisms have been reported. However, critical review of these reports to deduce a common ground for nongenotoxic carcinogenesis suggests that long-lasting epigenetic effects causing cell proliferation or sustained cellular hyperfunction/dysfunction may predispose to neoplastic transformation and therefore may act on their target sites as nongenotoxic carcinogens (Hayashi 1992).

It should be stressed that the toxicity test guidelines published in Japan include the following introductory note: “It is not always reasonable to apply a unified method for all chemicals, and therefore, the experimental methods noted here are not intended to be strictly followed as long as the data obtained are useful for safety evaluation of the test chemical in man.” This statement also is applicable to the highest-dose selection for carcinogenicity studies. Furthermore, there is a general consensus in the Japanese government that toxicity test guidelines, including carcinogenicity test guidelines, can be revised in accordance with recommendations of international bodies such as the ICH or in reflection of advances in areas of science and technology pertaining to toxicity evaluation. Revision of the scientific principles for highest dose selection in carcinogenicity testing is expected in the near future.

Dose Selection

Various guidelines (MHW 1984, MHW 1990, MAFF 1985, MHW 1988, MHW 1989) have commonly adopted the MTD principle as the standard method for highest-dose selection, in line with the requirements given in relevant publications of other countries or international bodies such as the United States, United Kingdom, Canada, the International Agency for Research on Cancer (IARC), or OECD. The definitions or criteria for defining the toxicity-based endpoint necessary for MTD determination tend to differ in some respects from guideline to guideline.

In addition to the MTD-based principle, Japanese guidelines also have described the MFD principle as an acceptable method for highest-dose selection, particularly for test chemicals with very weak toxicity.

Following are various definitions used by different Japanese regulatory authorities for the highest dose used in chronic animal bioassays:

> The dose in the preliminary carcinogenicity study that inhibits body weight gain by less than 10% in comparison with the control and causes neither death due to toxic effects nor remarkable changes in the general signs and laboratory examination findings of the animals is the highest dose to be used in the full-scale carcinogenicity study. (MHW 1984)

The carcinogenicity test guidelines for environmental chemicals enacted according to the Chemical Substances Control Law in Japan indicates that the highest-dose level is the maximum dose capable of causing slight depression of body-weight gain, no severe change in general conditions, or toxic death in preliminary short-term toxicity studies of 1 to 3 months duration (MHW 1990).

According to the test guidelines for agricultural chemicals, the highest test dose should be set at a level sufficiently high to elicit signs of minimal toxicity in animals (such as slight suppression of body-weight gain) without substantially altering the normal life span due to toxic effects other than tumor induction (MAFF 1985).

The MFD literally can be defined as the maximum practically or technically administrable dose in a particular route or mode of dosing. In the case of feeding studies, it has been stated that, to avoid excessive alteration of the nutritional balance of the diet, the test chemical should not constitute more than 5% of the diet.

An alternative method for high-dose selection for pharmaceuticals is "as an exception, it is also acceptable in cases where the test substance has a very low toxicity compared to the therapeutic dose in humans, to set the highest dose at about 100 times the clinical dose. In such cases it is necessary to indicate the justification for such a decision" (MHW 1989). However, this clinical dose-based principle recently has been deleted from the Japanese guidelines in accordance with the recommendations made at the First International Conference on Harmonization (MHW 1993).

It should be mentioned further that the MHW is now revising the section on dose selection in the current carcinogenicity test guidelines in consideration of the ICH harmonized tripartite guideline on dose selection for carcinogenicity studies of pharmaceuticals. The revisions state "This guidance outlines five generally acceptable criteria for selection of the high dose for carcinogenicity studies of therapeutics—maximum tolerated dose; 25-fold AUC [area under the curve] ratio (rodent/human); dose limiting pharmacodynamic effects; saturation of adsorption; and maximum feasible dose."

CANADA

Health Canada

Background

On 1 April 1995, Health Canada assumed responsibility for public health regulation of pesticides, pharmaceuticals, industrial chemicals, and food additives; it is the only agency in Canada responsible for human health risk assessment.

Health Canada uses the results of a chronic bioassay as a part of its weight-of-the-evidence approach to evaluate the carcinogenic potential of a chemical. But this approach means that the bioassay is only one item of a data package. A chemical that yields a positive result is one that generates a cancer incidence significantly above concurrent or historical control incidences in at least one sex of one species. However, positive results in both sexes of two species would be strong evidence toward the conclusion that the chemical was a carcinogen in the test species. Further, if epidemiological data do not suggest an association with cancer, if there is no structural similarity to known carcinogens, or if the chemical shows no genotoxicity, then the positive bioassay would be examined as described below.

There are numerous considerations taken into account when interpreting the results of a chronic bioassay. A chemical under certain conditions may increase the tumor incidence in an animal species, but that result may not be considered relevant to humans. The result may reflect species specificity or some other property of the model system. A weight-of-evidence approach is then required to interpret the data and allow regulators flexibility in their assessment of a chemical. A full assessment requires the consideration of certain biological factors. Consistent with Health Canada's examination of the results from chronic studies is a paper by Clayson et al. (1991), which states several of these factors, including the following:

Body Weight and Body Weight Gain
If the experimental group has a mean body weight gain that is 10% less than the control group, then this is considered a toxic effect. Severe decreases in body weight gain can impair the interpretation of the results. A decrease in weight gain due to poor food consumption may result in premature animal death or may even decrease the incidence of tumors because of decreased caloric intake.

Metabolism/Toxicokinetics/Toxicodynamics
If an animal's ability to metabolize a test chemical is unlike metabolism in humans, then the toxicity generated should be considered species-specific. In addition, if the animal's metabolic ability is saturated then the chemical may accumulate. This could result in a rise of the test chemical concentration in the blood. Bioaccumulation may lead to toxicity at other sites in the host.

Physiological Conditions
The test chemical may lead to altered pH values, osmolality, nucleotide pools, DNA replication or repair enzymes. Alteration of any of these parameters could enhance the likelihood of mutation and of cancer formation.

Species-Specific Considerations
In addition to metabolic aspects, certain species may demonstrate chemical-related carcinogenic effects, which may be species-specific and therefore not relevant to toxicity in humans. For example, male rats produce a protein, α_{2u}-globulin, which can combine with exogenous compounds and precipitate in the kidneys. The resulting nephropathy can subsequently develop into kidney cancer. There is no α_{2u}-globulin produced in female rats or in humans and, therefore, this mechanism is sex and species-specific.

Tissue-Specific Consideration
Most hormones have their effect on specific tissues. If a test chemical alters hormonal homeostasis then it could indirectly promote cancer development in a tissue specific manner. For example, ethylthiouracil interferes with the production of thyroid hormone. The result is an altered homeostasis, with a decrease of T_3 (triiodothyronine) in the blood and a subsequent increase in thyroid stimulating hormone. This stimulates cell division in the thyroid and in some animal models it can enhance cancer development.

Enhanced Cell Proliferation
Some chemicals can directly enhance cell division. Other chemicals can result in cell death and stimulate compensatory cell proliferation. In either

case, enhanced cell proliferation can increase the probability that a mutation will be fixed and that clonal expansion of the mutated cell will occur.

Structural Activity
If a test chemical has a structure not similar to known carcinogens, then a positive result may reflect one of the above considerations.

Incorporating these factors into the regulator's evaluation allows each chemical to be reviewed on an individual basis. The results of this approach yield a more scientifically credible conclusion and better protection for the public.

Dose Selection

Health Canada has no official guidelines on dose selection for chronic bioassays. However, this issue has been addressed in a 1991 Food Directorate publication (Health Canada 1991). It states:

> The difficulty in setting the highest dose level arises from the need to select a dose level that provides the highest probability of demonstrating tumors without shortening the lifespan or depressing the clinical condition of the test animal and at the same time, is the highest dose possible to fulfill these conditions.

The publication continues to explain:

> If the highest tolerated dose level is not used, there is the danger that the repetition of the study at a higher, but tolerated, dose level will give a positive result, whereas the original but lower level failed to do so.

Health Canada expects that a MTD would be used in chronic studies and its selection should include the following:

> (1) The selection for the maximum tolerated dose for chronic studies should be based on information derived from subchronic studies (e.g. 90-day study). These studies would include data on the sequential changes (if any) on body weight effects, clinical signs, diet consumed, hematology, urinalysis, clinical chemistry, pathology, and histology. Each of these parameters would be measured and examined often and thoroughly. Depending on the nature and severity of the changes observed, the highest dose tested for the chronic study may be a somewhat lower dose than the dose which induced significant changes in the 90-day study. An example of a significant change would be one that generated a statistically different value than the experimental control.
>
> (2) The highest dose selected for the chronic bioassay should not exceed 5% of the weight of the diet (50,000 ppm), or the maximum feasible dose.

(3) It is expected that the highest dose used for testing reflects the data derived from metabolism and toxicokinetic studies. Changes in the metabolic profile might occur with repeated exposure to the chemical or with very high doses of a chemical. A minor pathway might become significant with respect to the production of a toxic metabolite, as a consequence of bioaccumulation.

In addition to the MTD, at least two other doses are expected to be used in a chronic bioassay. The lowest dose used should not result in any toxicity or changes in growth, development, or longevity of the test animals. The intermediate dose may or may not evoke some minor toxicity. The doses do not have to be an exact fraction of the MTD. Ideally, they should be sufficiently different that they generate distinct toxicologic responses in the test animals.

Lastly, Health Canada realizes that the MTD is difficult to predict accurately. Animals do receive doses that exceed the MTD; positive results under those conditions require greater scrutiny in the risk-assessment process. Animals also receive doses below the MTD. Failure to reach the MTD does not automatically mean that a study is rejected and should be repeated. Historically, Health Canada has examined all of these MTD scenarios individually as one part of a complete data package. Ideally, the dose-selection process will incorporate the MTD, produce biologically credible results, and ensure scientifically defensible evaluations.

UNITED STATES

Environmental Protection Agency: Toxic Substances

Background

The Toxic Substances Control Act (TSCA) authorizes the Office of Pollution Prevention and Toxics (OPPT) within the U.S. Environmental Protection Agency (EPA) to restrict or prohibit the manufacture, processing, distribution, use, or disposal of chemical substances already in commerce and of new substances when there is a reasonable basis to conclude that any such activity poses an unreasonable risk to human health or the environment. If there is significant human or environmental exposure to a chemical or if the EPA suspects that a chemical substance may pose an unreasonable risk based on data for structurally related substances but lacks sufficient data to take action, Section 4 of TSCA empowers the agency to require the manufacturers and processors of such chemicals to develop the necessary data.

TSCA requires the EPA to consider and weigh 1) health and environmental risks, 2) potential costs and benefits, and 3) availability of alternative materials or technologies before taking any risk-reduction actions. The major approach taken by the OPPT for dealing with hazardous substances has two major levels of evaluation. At the initial screening level (i.e., risk- management level 1 [RM1]), readily available hazard and exposure data from reliable sources are reviewed to identify candidates for risk reduction. Qualitative judgments about the nature and magnitude of likely risk usually are made at this screening level. The next levels of evaluation (i.e., RM2 and post-RM2) entail a critical analysis of all relevant hazard and exposure data and an assessment of quantitative and qualitative expressions of risk.

For an in-depth evaluation of carcinogenic risk, the OPPT generally follows EPA's carcinogen risk-assessment guidelines, which employ a four-step process. 1) Hazard identification involves a qualitative review of all data bearing on the potential carcinogenicity of the chemical. The review culminates in a weight-of-the-evidence judgment of the likelihood that a chemical may be carcinogenic in humans. 2) Dose-response evaluation involves extrapolation of observed tumor findings in animal or human studies to predict potential carcinogenic effects at other, usually lower, doses of chemical exposure. In the absence of adequate mechanistic data, the OPPT generally employs the linearized multistage procedure to obtain an upper-limit risk estimate. 3) Exposure assessment identifies populations exposed to the agent and the physical and chemical form of the substance as well as the amount, frequencies, durations, and routes of exposure to the agent. The OPPT uses both measured and modeled data to predict an individual's exposure. 4) Risk characterization involves integrating the results of exposure and dose-response assessments to estimate quantitatively the carcinogenic risk.

There are several possible interpretations of the statistical and biological significance of the study and of the relevance of tumorigenic effects associated with exposure or dose levels below, at, or above the MTD. Positive studies at exposure or dose levels below or near the MTD usually are considered relevant for hazard identification and dose-response assessment. The absence of neoplastic effects in an adequately dosed study that has reached a MTD and is well-conducted is generally accepted as a negative finding. Studies with excessive dosing that show no tumors are accepted as negative if lower doses are appropriately spaced and mortality does not eliminate too many animals from the study. Studies that show tumors only at excessive doses are compromised and may or may not carry weight, depending on the interpretation in the context of other study results and other lines of evidence. Results of such studies, however, generally are not considered suitable for risk extrapolation.

In all cases, OPPT emphasizes the need for utilizing all pertinent data for a balanced conclusion regarding the carcinogenicity of the test substance. The overall interpretation of long-term carcinogenicity studies routinely considers results of long-term studies in conjunction with findings of subchronic studies, genotoxicity and other short-term tests, structure- activity relationships, comparative metabolism and toxicokinetic studies, and any other special studies.

EPA thus far has promulgated a number of test rules and negotiated consent orders under Section 4 of TSCA for carcinogenicity testing by inhalation or ingestion in rats and mice for 17 chemical substances. Only 11 substances have been or are being tested because six of the chemicals did not meet the triggered requirements. To date, the EPA has received test results for eight chemicals and has accepted all as adequate studies. Despite the lack of detailed guidance for dose selection, there has been virtually no disagreement among the test sponsors and OPPT concerning this issue and the adequacy of carcinogenicity testing for these substances. A continuing dialogue is believed to be a key reason for a generally good history with the test sponsors in meeting carcinogenicity testing requirements under TSCA.

Dose Selection

TSCA guidelines for carcinogenicity and combined chronic toxicity and carcinogenicity testing initially were developed in 1985, revised in 1987 and 1989 (EPA 1989), and harmonized with the equivalent Federal Insecticide, Fungicide, and Rodenticide Act (FIFRA) guidelines in 1995. The objective of long-term carcinogenesis bioassays under TSCA is to determine the carcinogenic potential and dose-response relationships of the test agents. TSCA test guidelines specify the use of at least three dose levels in addition to the concurrent control group. TSCA test guidelines provide only general guidance for selecting the doses. It is recommended that the selection generally be based on existing data, preferably on results of subchronic studies and toxicokinetic data if available. In practice, OPPT has always required subchronic toxicity testing if available data are not considered adequate for assessing systemic toxicity. Thus, dose selection for long-term carcinogenesis bioassays is always based on, at the minimum, findings of a subchronic 90-day study. Pharmacokinetic studies are required only in a few cases and occasionally are conducted voluntarily by the test sponsors to provide a more reliable data set for determining appropriate dosing for the bioassay.

The high-dose level should "...elicit signs of minimal toxicity without substantially altering the normal life span" (EPA 1989). The guidelines further specify the highest concentration for a diet mixture should not exceed 5%. The lowest dose should not induce any indications of toxicity, i.e., it should not interfere with normal growth, development, and longevity of the animal. The intermediate dose(s) should be established in a mid-range between the high and low doses. It also is stated in the guidelines that, in general, the low dose should not be lower than 10% of the high dose.

Although the term MTD is not explicitly used in TSCA carcinogenicity test guidelines, it generally is assumed that the high dose should be the MTD. As stated in the cancer risk assessment guidelines of the EPA, "long-term animal studies at or near the maximum tolerated dose level are used to ensure an adequate power for the detection of carcinogenic activity" (EPA 1986). The aim in dose selection is to achieve adequate sensitivity to determine whether the test substance has any carcinogenic potential and whether the observed tumorigenic response is specific to the test agent. Failure to reach an adequately high dose reduces the sensitivity of the study because the animals may not be sufficiently challenged. A lack of tumorigenic responses at exposure levels that cause significant impairment of animal survival also may not be acceptable as negative findings because of the reduced sensitivity of the study. On the other hand, excessive general toxicity in a target tissue for neoplastic effects raises the question of whether tumorigenic effects are specific to the agent or are nonspecific effects secondary to toxicity.

OPPT has not published any formal guidance concerning the definition of a MTD or criteria for determining whether a MTD has been reached or exceeded. In current practice, OPPT considers evidence of systemic toxicity to be the most critical factor in determining whether the administered dose has reached or exceeded the MTD. Examples of evidence of systemic toxicity include a 10% or greater increase in mortality as a result of toxicity and significant toxicity manifested by treatment-related changes in body-weight (gain of greater than 10%), clinical signs, hematology, clinical chemistry, and organ weight, morphology, and histopathology.

Currently, TSCA test guidelines do not define an upper-limit dose for inhalation and dermal studies. In practice, OPPT generally takes into consideration certain limiting factors in inhalation studies including the minimum oxygen content available to the animals (otherwise the test agent will act as an asphyxiant), the "overload" conditions of the respiratory system, and the explosive concentration of the test chemical. For dermal studies, skin toxicity is considered to be an important factor in defining the upper limit of the applied dose.

Environmental Protection Agency: Pesticides

Background

When carcinogenicity data are required under FIFRA, the same general principles of dose selection apply as stated above for TSCA. The Office of Pesticide Programs has the authority to require cancer bioassays to be conducted in at least two species, one of which is the rat. The mouse is most commonly used as the second species, although occasionally the hamster is used. The same testing guidelines apply under both TSCA and FIFRA. Although each office has the ability to require a subchronic study in the rat for the purpose of dose selection for the chronic study and other reasons, there is no guideline requirement for a similar study in the second species.

The Office of Pesticide Programs subjects virtually all environmental agents that are of interest to the EPA to the qualitative and quantitative assessment described below when data from the appropriate human epidemiologic studies or long-term animal carcinogenicity bioassays exist.

The Office of Pesticide Programs uses these data in two ways. The first is to provide a qualitative evaluation of the potential of the environmental agent of interest to produce a carcinogenic response in humans. It is well known that the EPA utilizes a five-category weight-of-evidence scheme to characterize its level of concern regarding likely human cancer potential. This weight-of-evidence scheme incorporates the evaluation of all pertinent long-term animal study results and human epidemiologic data as well as supporting data such as those on genotoxic effects, pharmacokinetics, and structure-activity relationships.

The second purpose for which the EPA uses data from long- term carcinogenicity bioassays is to perform dose-response evaluations and develop quantitative expressions of carcinogenic hazard to estimate excess carcinogenic risk. The EPA's Guidelines for Carcinogenic Risk Assessment (1986) describe the default principles and procedures used in the absence of chemical-specific, biologically relevant information. Two major factors are the assumptions that the carcinogenic response possesses no threshold of effect and that mathematical modeling of the dose-response is appropriate for calculating the chemical's potency expression. The greater the likelihood that an agent may be a human carcinogen, the greater the likelihood that these two assumptions will be applied in the risk assessment of that agent. Biologically relevant data, particularly on the mechanism(s) and mode(s) of action involved in the etiology of the observed tumor response, increasingly lead the EPA to use alternative quantitative methodologies that more accurately reflect the magnitude of risk.

Dose Selection

The FIFRA test guidelines require a minimum of three dose levels. However, no guidance is provided regarding selection of the lowest and intermediate levels.

Experience has taught the EPA and its regulated community that early consultation with regulatory scientists to discuss the design of a subacute/

subchronic repeated-dose study and use of the results to select doses for the chronic/carcinogenicity study reduce significantly the likelihood that the results from the long-term study will be rejected or "misused" when they are submitted to the EPA for review.

The Office of Pesticide Programs embraces the concept of the MTD in the design of studies to evaluate environmental agents for carcinogenic potential. Preferably, the MTD is a value derived from observed toxicities in subchronic studies conducted before the long-term study.

In the mid-1980s, the Toxicology Branch in the Office of Pesticide Programs issued a position document that described the criteria for selecting a MTD for the chronic study and for judging it to be achieved, exceeded, or underestimated in the long-term study: "the highest dose to be tested in the carcinogenicity study should elicit significant toxicity without substantially altering the normal life span of the test species" (EPA 1987).

In general, the principles espoused then continue to be applied today. But currently, as then, the definition of "significant" is not always agreed upon by all parties; thus, the principles may not always be consistently applied. Decrements of up to 10% in body-weight gain as well as biologically significant changes in the histologic, clinical chemistry, and hematologic profiles are phenomena that would indicate that a MTD was achieved. Organ-weight changes without significant attendant pathology would be interpreted as an indicator of inadequate dosing. In addition, a dose limit of 1000 mg/kg/day is considered to be an adequate upper limit for testing pesticides.

Food and Drug Administration: Pharmaceuticals

Background

Traditionally, carcinogenicity studies needed to support marketing of chronic-use pharmaceuticals within the United States have been designed, conducted, and interpreted according to the same principles established for other chemicals (Interagency Staff Group on Carcinogens 1986). Still, important distinctions may be made between pharmaceuticals and other chemicals that may influence study design and interpretation. For pharmaceuticals, there is usually an extensive database on human safety available from controlled clinical studies. Human exposures may be quite large (compared with environmental exposures), but they are intentional and definable. Perhaps most importantly, the benefit derived from using pharmaceuticals must be balanced with any risk associated with exposure.

Carcinogenicity studies are performed on pharmaceuticals primarily for hazard identification. Similar to other regulatory agencies, the Food and Drug Administration (FDA) uses a weight-of-evidence approach to interpret the outcome of carcinogenicity studies for pharmaceuticals. All relevant data are considered when the relevance of findings in rodents is assessed for human pharmaceutical use. In recent years, special emphasis has been placed on the value of mechanistic data for interpreting carcinogenicity study results, especially when increases in tumor incidence are thought to derive from mechanisms of questionable relevance for humans.

Decisions regarding marketing of pharmaceuticals with positive tumor findings are based on risk-benefit analyses, which consider the therapeutic indication, patient population, available alternative therapies, expected use patterns, duration of therapy, range of exposures, and human side effects along with the complete package of animal safety information (including carcinogenicity and genetic and reproductive toxicology data).

Dose Selection for Carcinogenicity Studies

To provide a maximum opportunity to detect a neoplastic response, regulatory agencies in the United States traditionally have recommended that the high dose in carcinogenicity studies represents the MTD. Consideration is given to a broad range of biological information in selecting the MTD, including alterations in body and organ weights; changes in hematologic, urinary, and clinical chemistry parameters; and the more definitive toxic, pathologic, and histopathologic endpoints. Traditionally, the middle and lowest doses chosen for testing in carcinogenicity studies have provided information on the shape of the dose-response curve and have ensured data for comparison with the control group when the high dose selected exceeded the MTD, especially when excessive mortality occurred in the high-dose group. Consideration of pharmacokinetic data has been encouraged when selecting low and middle doses, but historically such data rarely have been used. When available, pharmacokinetic data have been used primarily to demonstrate bioavailability or to justify routes or methods of administration other than those to be used in humans.

The development of increasing numbers of pharmaceuticals that showed little or no toxicity in rodent models created a problem for selecting a high dose in carcinogenicity studies based on toxicity alone. In some countries, a high multiple of the human dose was acceptable for dose selection for carcinogenicity studies of pharmaceuticals. However, as the justification for this arbitrary dose multiple was unclear, the FDA continued to require dosing to the MTD unless a MFD was used (e.g., 5% of diet).

In an effort to salvage carcinogenicity studies conducted at doses where no toxicity was observed, the Center for Drug Evaluation and Research Carcinogenicity Assessment Committee began requesting pharmacokinetic data that could give more realistic estimates of a safety margin than that given by dose multiples. When these data were used, some negative carcinogenicity studies were accepted to support regulatory approval, even when a MTD was not achieved, if a "high" margin of safety was indicated based on comparisons of rodent and human plasma areas under the curve (AUCs) or if saturation of absorption was demonstrated. The minimum acceptable margin of safety with this retrospective approach was determined on a case-by-case basis.

In 1992, the FDA began working with ICH to develop alternatives to the MTD for dose selection in carcinogenicity studies based on pharmacokinetic and pharmacodynamic considerations. To support a proposal for an alternative dosing strategy based on comparisons of systemic exposure, the FDA analyzed carcinogenicity studies performed at the MTD to determine what systemic exposure ratios were achieved in rodents at the MTD compared with humans using the maximum recommended daily dose.

Three important observations were made based on the database analysis performed: 1) a ratio of 25:1 is higher than that achieved by 75% of pharmaceuticals tested previously at the MTD; 2) use of a high dose representing a rodent-to-human AUC ratio of 25:1 in carcinogenicity studies would detect all pharmaceuticals previously classified as carcinogenic or probably carcinogenic to humans (IARC classifications 1 and 2A); and 3) relative doses (rodent to human) did not always predict relative systemic exposure margins. Thus, it was concluded that the overall testing stringency in carcinogenicity studies of pharmaceuticals was not lowered by accepting the AUC ratio of 25:1 as an endpoint for high-dose selection. On the basis of this analysis, an AUC ratio of 25:1 was accepted by ICH as providing an adequate margin of safety compared with human therapeutic exposure for nongenotoxic pharmaceuticals.

Dose Selection

Currently, the FDA accepts and endorses the dose-selection principles established in the ICH guideline "Dose Selection for Carcinogenicity Studies of Pharmaceuticals." Equally acceptable endpoints for the high-dose selection are the MTD, MFD, saturation of absorption, 25:1 AUC ratio, and dose-limiting pharmacodynamic effects. Other toxicity, pharmacokinetic, and pharmacodynamic endpoints may be considered for individual compounds based on scientific justification. The ICH document further delineates the general considerations the FDA endorses as important in selection of middle and low doses for carcinogenicity studies for pharmaceuticals. Such considerations include saturation of metabolic/detoxification pathways, use of doses producing the intended human therapeutic effect in the test species, nonlinearity of exposure with dose, and alterations in normal rodent physiology/hormone balance. All of these factors can influence the interpretation of the relevance of tumor findings for human use of pharmaceuticals, and factoring in these concerns when selecting middle and low doses is preferred to the standard practice of selecting arbitrary fractions of the high dose.

The Carcinogenicity Assessment Committee of the Center for Drug Evaluation and Research, in addition to providing a tertiary review of carcinogenicity study findings, also provides prospective guidance on dose selection. Under the investigational review process for new drugs, sponsors may seek agreement on proposed doses by submitting data that support their proposal. When adequate dose-range studies are available, and after review by Center for Drug Evaluation and Research staff, the sponsor receives concurrence on the doses selected or suggestions for alternative doses to be used in the chronic bioassay. This prospective agreement between the sponsor and the Carcinogenicity Assessment Committee on the adequacy of doses used in the bioassay eliminates a source of disagreement that otherwise can affect study acceptability. The acceptability of doses is determined in accordance with the ICH guidelines.

Food and Drug Administration: Food Additives

Background

This description of the basis for selection of doses to be used in the conduct of carcinogenicity studies for the FDA Center for Food Safety and Applied Nutrition (CFSAN) is modified from "Redbook II," the 1993 draft revision of the 1982 Redbook, also known as "Toxicological Principles for the Safety Assessment of Direct Food Additives and Color Additives Used in Food."

The CFSAN has appointed a multidisciplinary, centerwide committee, the Cancer Assessment Committee to provide an ongoing capability to analyze and interpret the results from chronic toxicity/carcinogenicity studies on food additives. The committee is composed of toxicologists, statisticians, chemists, pathologists, and epidemiologists. In addition, as circumstances warrant, scientists from other disciplines, including nutrition, may be invited to present data or provide interpretive expertise during the assessment of the carcinogenic potential of a food additive.

Typically, the Office of Premarket Approval, Division of Health Effects Evaluation, prepares a comprehensive analysis of present and previously conducted chronic toxicity/carcinogenicity studies on a specific food additive. This collection of data is reviewed by the Cancer Assessment Committee and an in-depth discussion of this and all other relevant information is undertaken. Among the elements that bear upon the findings of the Cancer Assessment Committee is whether there is a statistically significant increase in the incidence of tumors (the occurrence of benign and malignant tumors of a given type ordinarily are combined). However, only tumors of the same histologic origin are added together.

The Cancer Assessment Committee also considers other factors that may enhance the biological plausibility of a determination of carcinogenicity. Other factors considered include the site of other organ system toxicity and how it might contribute to the occurrence of organ-specific tumors and whether there are precursors of neoplasia, such as hyperplasia, in evidence. The Cancer Assessment Committee also considers and compares the incidence of compound-mediated tumors with the incidence of tumors and time of tumor onset in both concurrent and historic controls.

Another important consideration for the Cancer Assessment Committee is evidence for histopathologic diagnosis of specific tumor types. On selected occasions, it is necessary for the Office of Scientific Support, Pathology Branch, to ask petitioners for elaboration or clarification of the pathology results presented in a study. If the petitioner or sponsor for a study is unable to satisfactorily resolve questions surrounding the histopathologic diagnosis, then the Cancer Assessment Committee may formally request that the sponsor provide tissue microslides for the Pathology Branch so that the diagnosis presented by the sponsor of the food additive may be confirmed.

After careful consideration and evaluation of the data components discussed above, the Cancer Assessment Committee will conclude whether there are sufficient data to list the food additive as a carcinogen. On selected occasions, the Cancer Assessment Committee of the CFSAN may request that outside authorities in carcinogenic assessment (e.g., the Board of Scientific Counselors of the National Toxicology Program [NTP]) review its deliberation and conclusion regarding the carcinogenic potential of a food additive.

In most cases, once the Cancer Assessment Committee has determined that a compound is a carcinogen, that substance may not intentionally be added to food, unless the estimate of risk of carcinogenicity from exposure to a specified level of a carcinogenic constituent (impurity) is less than 10^{-6}, as determined from an appropriately conducted study by the Center's Quantitative Risk Assessment Committee. In the process of determining the risk estimate for a given carcinogen, the Cancer Assessment Committee reviews the quality and design of available studies to assess the carcinogenic potential of a food additive and selects the study that provides the best quality of information as the basis for the Quantitative Risk Assessment Committee's determination of that constituent's risk estimate.

Dose Selection

Carcinogenicity studies ordinarily are conducted in rodent species for 24 months, a major portion of their life span. Typically, data from previous subchronic studies are available to identify and support the selection of dose levels of the test substance; at least three dose levels are tested. The incidence of fatalities should not be so high or the time of the test so limited that a meaningful measure of the carcinogenic potential of the compound of interest is precluded.

Generally, it is not considered acceptable practice to base the highest dose administered on information unrelated to the toxicity of the material to be tested. For instance, it is not appropriate to use only a predetermined margin of safety above the projected maximum level of human exposure as the basis for specifying the highest dose to be tested. This is especially true if the dose results in no identifiable toxic response. The CFSAN recommends that the highest dose tested be the MTD. The CFSAN relies on the following definition of the MTD:

> that dose which, when given for the duration of the chronic study as the highest dose, will not shorten the treated animals' longevity from any toxic effects other than the induction of neoplasms (Sontag et al. 1976).

Thus, the CFSAN's interpretation of this definition is that the highest possible dose of the test material should be administered to the test animals so long as they do not die prematurely of any toxic endpoint except as caused by compound-induced neoplasms. On the other hand, the MTD should not produce any morphologic alterations of such severity that they interfere with or obscure the interpretation of the study.

As time has passed and experience with carcinogenicity testing has accumulated, it has become more apparent that information from a greater breadth of physiologic indicators can be used to assist in the selection of the MTD. Therefore, in addition to the more traditional indicators, such as body and organ weight changes and gross or histopathologic modifications, clinically significant alterations of hematologic, urinary, and clinical chemistry measurements also may be integrated into the determination of the MTD.

The high dose for the chronic toxicity study generally lies between the dose level that causes a positive endpoint and the dose that has a minimal effect in the 90-day test (NTP 1984). One series of findings usually interpreted to indicate a positive or toxic endpoint is the manifestation of moderate to marked necrosis, degeneration, irritation, inflammation, or atrophy of an organ. Further support for the interpretation of a positive effect is provided by a specific lesion observed to occur in a dose-responsive manner and for which no evidence is found in the control group of test animals.

The NTP (1984) describes the possibility of compound-induced changes in the weight of certain organs that may be observed before the identification of specific lesions in these organs. Moreover, changes in body weight may be even more sensitive and indicate effects that are not otherwise apparent. The aforementioned changes may, in appropriate circumstances, represent toxic endpoints. It should be noted, however, that convincing data (perhaps some type of independently manifested evidence) and scientific logic would have to be presented to allow the CFSAN to use this type of relatively subtle toxic effect to be interpreted as an indication that the MTD had been achieved.

Clinical laboratory measurements often are performed during 90-day studies to assess whether multidose exposure to the test material has produced adverse responses in hematologic, clinical chemistry, or urinary components. Routine clinical chemistry assessment is commonly less sensitive in detecting compound- mediated adverse effects than are measurements of organ weights or histopathologic analyses of organ systems. It is appropriate to analyze urine volume, specific gravity, and microscopic urine sediment when renal toxicity is probable or suspected. Hematologic tests are a reasonable method of identifying toxic changes in the hematopoietic system. A more complete discussion of the strengths and limitations of this type of data in assessing the toxic potential of the test material is provided in NTP (1984).

The incidence of mortality induced by the test material in a 90-day study is monitored and, if increased, serves as an indicator of the need for reassessing the dosage levels used in the study. Most subchronic studies also plan for daily and careful observation of the test animals for signs of clinical effects. Certain kinds of clinical effects (e.g., profound sedation or anesthesia) may indicate the need to lower the dose administered.

The CFSAN understands that its recommendation to conduct carcinogenicity studies at the MTD carries with it the possibility of dosage administration so high that inappropriate or unrepresentative effects may be elicited. If, for example, histopathologic damage is so severe in an organ or tissue being evaluated for neoplastic response that diagnosis becomes compromised or impossible, then results from a lower-dosed group of animals may be required. Using examples of experimental findings of this nature and other previously described observations as a basis, CFSAN is considering alternative approaches to the selection of maximum doses; however, at the present time, there is no accepted alternative to the use of the MTD (as determined in the traditional manner) in studies being performed to assess the carcinogenic potential of a food additive.

It is quite useful for the CFSAN petitioner to provide a discussion in the final study report of how the highest dose was selected. Even with the results of a properly conducted subchronic study, however, the CFSAN recognizes that determination of the MTD is no more than an estimate of toxicity; during the course of the chronic study, the extension or intensification of toxic effects can render the results of the highest dose tested difficult to interpret.

The Redbook II also provides guidance in the selection of other doses that are administered in the carcinogenic study. With respect to the determination of the lowest dose, it should not interfere with normal growth, development, and life span of the test animals, nor should it produce any other signs of toxicity. Generally speaking, however, the lowest dose should not be less than 10% of the highest dose. The intermediate dose may be selected on the basis of the pharmacokinetic properties of the test material.

In certain studies, an optional fourth dose may be given as well. For example, if significant differences exist in the pharmacokinetic or metabolic profiles of the test substance given at the highest and lowest doses, a fourth dose level may be included in the study. In this particular case, the optional dose level should be selected to elicit the same or similar pharmacokinetic or metabolic effects as those obtained at the lowest dose. It is preferable to include extra animals at this test dose so that the approximate sensitivity to detect a carcinogenic response is the same as in the highest dose group tested.

Public Health Service: National Institute for Environmental Health Sciences, National Toxicology Program

Background

The selection of doses for the rodent carcinogenicity studies performed by the NTP traditionally has been conducted according to guidelines set forth by national and international advisory groups (Sontag et al. 1976, National Research Council 1977, IARC 1980, NTP Board of Scientific Counselors 1984, Office of Science and Technology Policy 1985, McConnell et al. 1989, NRC 1993). These groups have considered and accepted the premise that laboratory animal studies for carcinogenesis must use doses that exceed those associated with most human exposures to compensate for the small population of test animals used as surrogates for the human population.

In partial fulfillment of its mission to provide information on potentially toxic substances, the NTP publishes a Technical Report series on the results of NTP-sponsored toxicology and carcinogenesis studies in rodents. In addition, the NTP is required by Public Law 95-622 to publish a report on carcinogens for information purposes. Neither document series is a regulatory instrument or is in any way legally binding.

The reporting of a chemical as a carcinogen in either the Technical Report or the Biennial Report on Carcinogens series is considered the first step in hazard identification. The listings are qualitative in nature and form only part of the total risk-assessment process. In the Technical Reports, chemicals are assigned a level of evidence of carcinogenic activity (no, equivocal, some, clear, or inadequate study) based on an evaluation of the strength of the carcinogenic response under the conditions of the assay. The potential human health significance of the findings is addressed in the discussion sections of these documents when possible, but identification of a substance as a carcinogen is based solely on the findings in rodents.

In the biennial reports, substances are identified for inclusion primarily from the NTP Technical Reports or from working groups of the International Agency for Research on Cancer. Both human and animal studies are used to identify chemicals as possible carcinogens in humans. Substances are placed into one of three categories:

- substances or groups of substances and medical treatments that are known to be carcinogenic;
- substances or groups of substances and medical treatments that may reasonably be anticipated to be carcinogens;
- occupational exposures associated with a technological process that are known to be carcinogenic.

Known carcinogens are defined as those substances for which the evidence from human studies indicates there is a causal relationship between exposure to the substance and human cancer. Substances "which may reasonably be anticipated to be carcinogens" are defined as those for which there is limited evidence of carcinogenicity in humans or sufficient evidence of carcinogenicity in experimental animals. Sufficient evidence in animals is demonstrated by positive carcinogenicity findings in multiple strains and species of animals, in multiple experiments, or to an unusual degree with regard to incidence, site, type of tumor, or age at onset.

Dose Selection

The NTP conducted prechronic and 2-year rodent bioassays on nearly 500 chemicals and has considered a variety of factors in selection of the highest dose for the 2-year rodent studies. To illustrate the factors that have influenced selection of the highest dose in NTP 2-year bioassays, information on dose selection was gathered from 2-year NTP studies that began after 1 January 1985. Not all of the 2-year studies conducted during this time provided useful information. For example, studies evaluating several gavage vehicles used preset limited volumes and were not preceded by prechronic studies (NTP 1993a). Other studies evaluated the effect of perinatal versus adult-only exposure or explored lower reaches of dose-response curves for known carcinogens (NTP 1993b, 1993c). Thus, a total of 79 studies provided useful prechronic study information, 49 of which have been completed and reviewed as technical reports by the NTP Board of Scientific Councilors Peer Review Subcommittee as of November 1994.

Table 3 shows the number of groups (sex/species) evaluated and the studies categorized according to route of administration and completion. Table 4 shows the number of groups for which mortality, body-weight gains, or pathology in critical target organs was considered the single most important

Table 3. NTP 2-year study data set, 1984 to 1994

Route	Experimental groups	Chemicals	Completed technical reports
Gavage	62	17	11
Feed	88	23	16
Drinking Water	26	8	5
Inhalation	82	21	5
Dermal	38	10	4
Totals	**296**	**79**	**44**

Table 4. Critical factors or target organs for dose selection for all routes of exposure

	Experimental groups by exposure route					Total by	
Factor or target organ	Gavage	Feed	Drinking water	Inhalation	Dermal	experimental groups	Total by chemicals
Body Weight	10	26	13	12		61	20
Other	2	18	2	6	8	36	12
Mortality	19	2	1	4		26	11
Liver	8	14	2	2		26	10
Skin					30	30	8
Lung	2			20		22	6
Kidney	9	6	2	4		21	8
Bone marrow/ blood	6	6		4		16	6
Nasal cavity				10		10	3
Clinical signs		6		4		10	3
Pharmaco-kinetics		4		4		8	2
Stomach	2		2	2		6	3
Larynx				4		4	1
Lung burden				4		4	1
Nervous System		2		2		4	2
Pancreas			4			4	1
Adrenal		2				2	1
Thyroid	2					2	1
Cardiovascular	2					2	1
Rectum		2				2	1
Total	62	88	26	82	38	**296**	**101**[a]

[a] Exceeds the total number of 79 chemicals because more than one factor often was critical in dose selection in the four sex/species combinations which comprised most single chemical studies.

limiting factor in the prechronic studies that determined the upper dose for the chronic studies.

Whenever possible, the MTD (after Sontag et al. 1976, NTP 1984, and Haseman and Lockhart 1994; also referred to as the minimally toxic dose after Huff et al. 1994) has been used in chronic exposure studies conducted by

NTP to ensure an adequate chemical challenge to the animals. The highest dose has been defined typically as "the highest dose of the test agent that can be predicted not to alter the animals' normal longevity from effects other than carcinogenicity" (NTP 1984). However, in practice, the criteria to select the highest dose have evolved over the years by virtue of the experience gained from the numerous studies conducted and reported by the NTP.

The route of administration for a study frequently influenced which factors were critical for dose selection. When the chemical was administered by gavage (Table 4), typically in corn oil, 19 of the sex/species groups evaluated showed no effects other than mortality in prechronic studies that were considered of sufficient biological importance to preclude the use of the particular dose level in chronic studies. When mortality was the limiting factor, doses selected for the 2-year studies ranged from 25% to 70% of the lethal dose depending on the bioaccumulative properties of the chemical and the appreciation for the cause of death. For example, doses closer to lethal levels have been successfully used for certain pharmaceuticals when the slope of the dose-response curve for pharmacologic action is steep and the pharmacologic action is the cause of death.

The data in Table 4 suggest that body-weight changes were the most common factor used in dose selection for chronic studies performed by the drinking-water and dosed-feed routes. Differential body-weight gains between dosed and control groups remain a primary endpoint on which to base chronic study dose selections. In the absence of discernible target organ histopathology or mortality, a decrease in weight gain of about 10% or more when compared to controls in 13-week studies or longer has been considered sufficient to eliminate a dose from consideration for a chronic study. However, there are many examples of instances when the ultimate effects on body-weight gains could not be predicted from the prechronic studies (NTP 1993a); weight effects often have stabilized by 13 weeks, and the patterns hold during longer studies. In general, body-weight effects in rats are more predictable and reproducible than in mice.

Inhalation studies of vapors and particularly of relatively insoluble particulates (talc, mineral fibers, diesel particulates, etc.) may provide the greatest challenge to dose (exposure concentration) selection because of the range of histopathologic effects produced in the respiratory system. Lung-burden information often is collected in prechronic studies for inhaled metals or other particulates but infrequently has proved to be the critical factor in dose selection for this small subset of NTP chemicals. The data in Table 4 suggest that target organ lesions in the lung, larynx, and nasal cavity are most often pivotal in prechronic studies by this route of exposure.

For dermal studies, systemic toxicity associated with chemical administration was not critical in dose selection for these chemicals (Table 4). Hyperplasia, hyperkeratosis, and inflammation at the site of application were the most commonly encountered lesions in prechronic studies. "Other" factors typically included a variety of technical or practical factors that limited the amount of chemical that could be delivered to an animal. For dermal studies, this frequently was the amount of chemical that could be administered in a maximum dermal application volume (0.3 ml for rats or 0.1 ml for mice). For feed studies, a 5% limit, by weight, of chemical in the diet was occasionally a practical limit; poor palatability of dosed-feed or drinking-water solutions was also a limiting factor.

An unusual pancreatic lesion composed of acinar cell degeneration and fatty change occurred in all four sex/species groups in the chloropropanol prechronic studies, and dose levels for the chronic study were set below those that resulted in the lesion. Similar situations, in which infrequently encountered lesions were critical in dose selection, included the finding of polyarteritis in the gavage studies of theophylline and rectal inflammation with diaminostilbene disulfonic acid (NTP 1992). These rather unique cases require the professional judgment of pathologists and toxicologists for proper dose selection.

It is evident from the data presented in Table 4 that the critical factors for dose selection vary according to the route of administration. Body-weight effects, local exposure reactions or effects, and practical considerations are the most frequently used determinants, although mortality and lesions of the liver, skin, respiratory tract, and kidney also have frequently influenced dose selection for chronic bioassays. Additional information derived from prechronic studies addressing clinical pathology, toxicokinetics, and cell proliferation also can influence dose selection for chronic rodent bioassays. Some of these issues are discussed briefly below and in greater detail in Chapter 5.

Clinical Pathology. The NTP experience with clinical pathology findings is the subject of a recent review (Travlos et al. 1996). Although clinical chemistry is a routine part of nearly every set of prechronic studies, the findings generally are not a factor in high-dose selection. Frequently, changes in serum enzymes indicative of liver toxicity are noted at dose levels lower than those that show evidence of histopathologic lesions. These findings are very useful for identifying NOAELs, but in no case has this degree of toxic response been considered sufficient to affect the life span of animals being tested, nor are these minor changes often associated with discernible effects on body weight; thus, doses showing only minor changes in clinical chemistry have been considered appropriate for use in a 2-year study.

In contrast, hematologic findings have been limiting in several instances and are indicated in Table 4 in the bone marrow/blood category. A recent example was the selection of a top exposure concentration for a 2-year inhalation study of 2- butoxyethanol that caused no more than a 15% change in hematologic indices indicative of a regenerative anemia (Chapin et al. 1994).

Chemical Metabolism, Disposition, and Kinetic Information. A second large body of data that only occasionally has been used in dose selection is information from studies of chemical disposition and metabolism. This information generally has been more useful in study interpretation, in determination of relevance of results to humans, and in comparisons of species and sex differences in toxicity and carcinogenicity. More recently, toxicokinetic studies have been included in selected prechronic and chronic studies; however, these findings have not yet had a major influence on dose selection. There are only two instances in the NTP database where toxicokinetic information has been crucial in dose selection. In selection of the concentrations for isobutene in a 2-year inhalation study, there were no lesions or changes in body-weight gains in prechronic studies that were considered of sufficient biological importance on which to base dose selection. Although the highest exposure concentration was set at 50% the flammable vapor concentration (a practical limit), the lower concentrations were selected on the basis of metabolic saturation and are discussed further under the sections on selection of middle and lowest doses.

An emerging approach at NTP is to use toxicokinetic data to select the highest dose in conjunction with other prechronic study findings. When considering a chemical showing nonlinear or biphasic elimination kinetics, if other factors permit, the highest dose for 2-year studies may be set above the inflection point in the "saturated" range. Middle and lower doses are selected in linear regions of the dose-response curve and are discussed further below.

It is possible that an expanded use of toxicokinetic information will not markedly affect dose selection for chronic studies insofar as toxicity, which would otherwise limit dose selection, may be expected to correspond with doses that exhibit "saturated" elimination kinetics. Conversely, when no evidence of toxicity is manifest under saturated conditions, there may be no a priori reason to avoid use of doses in the saturated range, especially if there is evidence of high exposure in humans.

Rate of Cell Proliferation (Organ Specific). This same general approach also is applicable to other information that has not traditionally been used in dose selection. For example, it is becoming increasingly common to determine estimates of the rates of cell proliferation in target organs as part of the prechronic study data set. There is general agreement that increased cell proliferation is a potentially strong risk factor for carcinogenesis in certain organs of selected species. Because there is a virtual absence of information on the dose response for cell proliferation in humans, it may be prudent to select doses that do and that do not cause increased cell proliferation in both 90-day and 2-year studies.

Histopathology Evidence. A general principle of dose selection based on histopathologic lesions is that the site, morphology, and severity of the treatment-related effects present at the highest dose should not adversely affect survival in a 2-year study. Treatment-related histopathologic lesions have been identified at more than 35 sites/tissues in rats and mice from NTP prechronic studies. The following section includes only the more common sites for histopathologic lesions that have occurred in NTP prechronic toxicity studies. It is recognized that important effects in the central and peripheral nervous, cardiovascular, endocrine, and reproductive systems as well as other sites are not included in the brief summary provided here. A general overview of lesions in the liver, gastrointestinal tract, kidney, respiratory tract, skin, and spleen/bone marrow/blood, which have been critical in dose selection for NTP carcinogenicity studies, follows.

Liver. Common treatment-related liver lesions include hypertrophy, necrosis and inflammation, bile duct or oval cell hyperplasia, cytoplasmic vacuolization/degeneration of hepatocytes, and pigment accumulation in Kupffer cells or hepatocytes. Minimal to mild hypertrophy or pigmentation frequently is present at doses selected for chronic studies. The presence of hepatocellular necrosis and inflammation, cytoplasmic vacuolization/degeneration, and bile duct or oval cell hyperplasia generally is considered to preclude selection of a dose for chronic study.

Gastrointestinal tract. In the gastrointestinal tract, treatment-related lesions important in dose selection generally have been limited to the forestomach. Minimal hyperplasia of the squamous epithelium, focal or diffuse in distribution, generally is considered to be a treatment effect that would not adversely affect growth and survival. However, more severe hyperplasia as well as inflammation, erosion, ulceration, or necrosis of the squamous epithelium are lesions that preclude selection of doses for a chronic study. Intestinal lesions were important in one study in which the maximum dose selected was below that which resulted in acute inflammation and erosion of the intestinal mucosa at the anorectal junction.

Kidney/urinary bladder. A number of treatment-related lesions that commonly occur in the kidney include exacerbation of nephropathy with increased severity of regeneration, fibrosis, and inflammation; hyaline droplet nephropathy, renal papillary degeneration (edema); papillary necrosis; and karyomegaly or pigmentation of renal tubule epithelium. Karyomegaly, pigmentation, papillary edema, and urinary bladder lesions (including minimal hyperplasia or pigmentation of the transitional epithelium) generally are minimal changes that do not limit dose selection. Occasionally, a maximum dose may be selected that causes a very slight increase over the minimal severity grade of spontaneous nephropathy normally seen in control rats. This increased severity of nephropathy is associated not with obvious necrosis of tubule epithelium or dilated renal tubules containing protein casts but rather with only a slight increase in the number of regenerative renal tubules.

Papillary necrosis and hyaline droplet nephropathy associated with necrosis and protein or granular cast formation in renal tubules are treatment-related effects that would preclude selection of doses for chronic studies. The presence of grossly visible calculi, more severe grades of hyperplasia or inflammation, and squamous metaplasia and/or necrosis and erosion of the urinary bladder mucosa are also treatment-related findings that would preclude selection of doses for a chronic study.

Respiratory system. Treatment-related lesions in inhalation studies commonly occur in the nasal passages, larynx, and/or lungs. Lesions in the nasal cavity include inflammation, necrosis, degeneration, hyperplasia, and metaplasia of the respiratory or olfactory epithelium.

In the nasal passages, hyperplasia, metaplasia (squamous or respiratory), degeneration (olfactory), and minimal to mild inflammation have not been limiting factors for dose selection. Lesions in the larynx commonly include degeneration, inflammation, and squamous metaplasia, which are characteristically subtle, minimal lesions that have not been factors in dose selection. Common treatment-related lesions in the lung include histiocytosis; acute inflammatory exudate within alveoli; interstitial inflammation and fibrosis; hyperplasia of alveolar type 2 cells; and hyperplasia, necrosis metaplasia, and karyomegaly of bronchiolar epithelium. Minimal histiocytosis and in some instances very minimal focal interstitial inflammation and fibrosis of alveolar septae have been present in doses selected for chronic study. Alveolar macrophages containing pigment granules from inhaled particulates and minimal karyomegaly or hyperplasia of bronchiolar or alveolar epithelium also have been included in doses selected for chronic study.

Necrosis and extensive acute inflammation with exudate within the lumen of the nasal passages have been limiting factors in selection of a maximum dose for a 2-year study. Inflammation with squamous metaplasia and hyperkeratosis in the anterior portion of the nose in mice has been a limiting factor related to potentially fatal obstruction of the nasal passages. Moderate necrosis and acute inflammation of the laryngeal mucosa with subsequent formation of large, potentially obstructive inflammatory polyps were a limiting factor in dose selection for one study. Necrosis with squamous metaplasia, extensive inflammation including granuloma formation, and acute inflammatory cell exudates within alveoli have not been features included in doses selected for chronic study.

Skin. Treatment-related lesions in the skin that have been limiting factors for dose selection have occurred only in dermal studies. Typical skin lesions include hyperplasia (acanthosis) of the stratum spinosum, hyperkeratosis, inflammation in the dermis and epidermis, necrosis or ulceration of the epidermis, and hypertrophy or hyperplasia of the sebaceous glands. Minimal to mild hyperplasia of the squamous epithelium, hyperkeratosis, and sebaceous gland hypertrophy or hyperplasia are effects present at maximum doses selected for chronic studies. Very minimal mononuclear inflammatory cell infiltrates within the dermis also are sometimes present. Limiting factors for dose selection have included more severe inflammation, necrosis, and ulceration of the epidermis.

Spleen/bone marrow/blood. Alterations in the hematopoietic system that are severe enough to be a critical factor for dose selection are not common. In most instances, changes such as hyperplasia in regional lymph nodes, spleen, or bone marrow are secondary effects representing a response to treatment-related lesions at other sites (inhaled particulates, erythrocyte destruction, skin erosions). Frequently, the primary toxic effects occurring at other sites or factors related to body- weight gain and mortality are more critical for dose selection. Treatment-related effects including minimal to mild increases in hematopoiesis, hemosiderin accumulation or depletion in the spleen, fibrosis, or congestion relative to that observed in controls may be present in doses selected for chronic study. Findings that are not generally considered acceptable for inclusion in a minimum toxic dose include necrosis and cellular depletion of bone marrow or hematologic evidence of a nonregenerative anemia.

ORGANIZATION FOR ECONOMIC COOPERATION AND DEVELOPMENT

Background

An essential aspect of the OECD is that this organization is not a supranational organization but rather a center for discussion where governments express their points of view, share their experiences, and search for common ground. This arrangement implies that decisions are made by consensus. Once the council, which is the highest authority of the OECD, adopts a formal decision, such a decision is binding on all member countries.

The OECD test guidelines form an integrated part of such a binding council decision. The same Council decision further states that: "Data generated in the testing of chemicals in an OECD member country in accordance with OECD Test Guidelines and OECD Principles of Good Laboratory Practice shall be accepted in other member countries for purposes of assessment and other use relating to the protection of man and the environment." This council decision usually is referred to as the mutual acceptance of data decision.

The current procedure involves nominating experts from all member countries to develop guideline proposals. Proposals are widely circulated for review before they are adopted. In addition, workshops and meetings among the experts are routinely used to reach consensus on all technical issues. However, in the late 1970s when the guidelines on carcinogenicity were developed, proposals were drafted by a "Group of Experts on Short Term and Long Term Toxicity." This group was composed of 56 experts from 13 member countries and the CEC. A considerable number of these experts attended only part of the meetings on carcinogenicity testing.

Historically, the concept of dose-level selection, which also was adopted by the OECD expert group, included maximizing exposure with an emphasis on carcinogenic potential in a qualitative sense. This concept seems to have gradually changed over the years to a more mechanistic approach with an emphasis on dose-response relationships. The national coordinators of the OECD Test Guidelines Programme agreed in 1994 that it is timely to revise and update the OECD test guidelines on carcinogenicity testing.

Dose Selection

In OECD Test Guidelines 451 (Carcinogenicity Studies) and 453 (Combined Chronic Toxicity/Carcinogenicity Studies), both adopted in May 1981, guidance on the selection of the highest dose is the following:

> The highest dose level should be sufficiently high as to elicit signs of minimal toxicity without substantially altering the normal life span due to effects other than tumors.

With respect to what constitutes "signs of minimal toxicity," the relevant OECD guidelines further state:

> Signs of toxicity are those that may be indicated by alterations in certain serum enzyme levels or slight depression of body weight gain (less than 10 percent).

Selection of other doses is guided by the following language:

> The lowest dose should not interfere with normal growth, development, and longevity of the animal; and it must not otherwise cause any indication of toxicity. In general this should not be lower than 10% of the high dose. The intermediate dose(s) should be established in a mid-range between the high and low doses, depending upon the toxicokinetic properties of the chemical, if known.

INTERNATIONAL CONFERENCE ON HARMONIZATION (1995)

Background

The First International Conference on Harmonization (ICH-1) was held in 1991. At that time, the following recommendations were made regarding the selection of high doses: 1) the criteria for dose selection for carcinogenicity studies should be neither the MTD nor an arbitrary multiple of the intended human dose; 2) dose selection should be accomplished by considering exposure levels in the test species and in humans; and 3) a working guideline should be developed for rational selection of appropriate exposures and the corresponding doses.

The Second International Conference on Harmonization was held in Orlando, Florida, in 1993. At that meeting, a consensus draft guideline (step 2 of the ICH process) was adopted regarding selection of doses for carcinogenicity studies of pharmaceuticals. The guideline, with some modification, was later approved as a final guidance (step 5 of the ICH process) and is being applied in all the signatory regions. The guideline proposes the use of any one of five approaches to determine the high-dose selection for carcinogenicity tests in rodents. These approaches are based on 1) toxicity-based endpoints, 2) pharmacokinetic endpoints, 3) saturation of absorption, 4) pharmacodynamic endpoints, and 5) the MFD. It also is recognized that, based on scientific rationale for an individual drug, there may be merit in the use of endpoints not specifically defined in the guidelines. Guidance also is provided for the determination of low and middle doses. The guidance emphasizes the need to use scientifically rational approaches to choose not only the high dose but also the middle and low doses for carcinogenicity studies. Selection of all dose levels should be undertaken while considering as much information as possible about the pharmacology, toxicology, and pharmacokinetics of the drug in both rodents and humans. Such an approach allows for the most scientifically rigorous interpretation of the study findings and aids in assessing potential human risk.

Dose Selection

Toxicity-Based Endpoints

Although it was originally proposed at ICH-1 that the MTD not be retained as a method for dose selection, the final guidance allows continued use of this endpoint as an appropriate toxicity-based endpoint for the selection of the highest dose. Other toxicity-based endpoints were not adopted, as there is no scientific consensus on their use for high-dose selection. The ICH guidance defines the MTD as follows:

> The top dose or maximum tolerated dose is that which is predicted to produce a minimum toxic effect over the course of the carcinogenicity study. Such an effect may be predicted from a 90-day dose range-finding study in which minimal toxicity is observed. Factors to consider are alterations in physiological function which would be predicted to alter the animal's normal life span or interfere with interpretation of the study. Such factors include: no more than 10% decrease in body weight gain relative to controls; target organ toxicity; significant alterations in clinical pathological parameters.

It should be noted that analysis of the FDA database on carcinogenicity studies conducted at the MTD (Contrera et al. 1995) indicated that about one-third of studies achieved a MTD at exposures lower than those achieved in humans during clinical use. Thus, in many cases, use of the MTD as an endpoint for high-dose selection does not result in "excessive dosing" in relation to human exposure.

Pharmacokinetic Endpoints

At ICH-1 it was concluded that an exposure-based endpoint should be developed for dose selection. It was recognized that because of differences in metabolism and drug disposition, "comparability of systemic exposure is better assessed by blood concentrations of parent drug and metabolites than by administered dose. The unbound drug in plasma is thought to be the most relevant indirect measure of tissue concentrations of unbound drug. The AUC is considered the most comprehensive kinetic endpoint since it takes into account the plasma concentration of the compound and residence time in vivo" (ICH 1995). Thus, it also was concluded that the pharmacokinetic endpoint should be based on achieving an AUC in rodents that was several times the exposure achieved in humans at the maximum recommended daily dose of the drug.

Three factors were considered paramount in selection of a relative systemic exposure ratio (AUC ratio to apply in high-dose selection): 1) that it represent an adequate margin of safety, 2) that it could be attained by a reasonable proportion of compounds, and 3) that its application would allow detection of known or probable human carcinogens.

To address these factors, the FDA's database on carcinogenicity studies was analyzed (Contrera et al 1995). This database is composed of 35 drug carcinogenicity studies conducted at the MTD for which there are adequate pharmacokinetic data in rats and humans. There was a relative systemic exposure ratio of the rodent MTD and the human maximum recommended daily dose of 1 for approximately one-third of the 35 drugs, a ratio between 1 and 10 for approximately one-third of the drugs, and a ratio exceeding 10 for approximately one-third of the drugs.

A 25× AUC was selected for the pharmacokinetic endpoint. The 25× ratio allows an adequate margin of safety compared with human therapeutic exposure and ensures that overall testing stringency in carcinogenicity studies of pharmaceuticals is not lowered with regard to relative rodent/human systemic exposures. The 25× AUC was achieved in about 25% of the pharmaceuticals tested previously at the MTD. Finally, use of a high dose representing a 25× rodent/human AUC in carcinogenicity would detect all pharmaceuticals previously classified as carcinogenic or probably carcinogenic to humans (IARC classification 1 or 2A) based on currently available information on an analysis of exposure or dose ratios (Contrera et al. 1995).

The ICH concluded that, although there is not a validated scientific basis for use of comparative drug plasma concentrations for the assessment of carcinogenic risk to humans, a dose that results in an AUC of the parent compound (or metabolites) in rodents that is 25 times (or greater) the human AUC at the maximum recommended human daily dose is acceptable for nongenotoxic substances. The ICH guidance lists the following criteria that are applicable for use of a pharmacokinetically defined exposure for high-dose selection:

1) Rodent pharmacokinetic data are derived from the strains used for the carcinogenicity studies with the route of compound administration and dose ranges planned for the carcinogenicity study.
2) Pharmacokinetic data are derived from studies of sufficient duration to take into account potential time-dependent changes in pharmacokinetic parameters that may occur during the dose-ranging studies.
3) Documentation is provided on the similarity of exposure of rodents and humans to the parent compound and metabolites. It is recommended that, if possible, in vivo metabolism be characterized in humans and rodents. However, in the absence of appropriate in vivo metabolism data, in vitro metabolism data (e.g., from liver slices, uninduced microsomal preparations) may provide adequate support for the similarity of metabolism across species.
4) In assessing exposure, scientific judgement is used to determine whether the AUC comparison is based on data for the parent, parent and metabolite(s), or metabolite(s). The justification for this decision should be provided.
5) Interspecies differences in protein binding are taken into consideration when estimating relative exposure.
6) Human pharmacokinetic data are derived from studies encompassing the human maximum recommended daily dose.

Saturation of Absorption

Nonlinearity in the pharmacokinetics of a drug was considered an important element in selection of doses for carcinogenicity studies. ICH (1995) guidance recommends that saturation of absorption measured by systemic availability of drug-related substances is acceptable for selection of the high dose. Saturation of metabolic and elimination pathways was felt to be of primary utility in selection of the middle and low doses for the carcinogenicity study and in interpretation of study findings, but it was not recommended as a high-dose selection endpoint.

Pharmacodynamic Endpoints

Pharmaceuticals often are developed on the basis of their receptor selectivity and the resultant pharmacodynamic effects. Because these properties often are identified initially on the basis of results from rodent models, rodents treated at high doses may exhibit pharmacodynamic effects that limit dose escalation. The types of responses produced will be highly compound specific and their use in selection of the high dose for carcinogenicity studies is considered on an individual basis according to scientific merit. The ICH guidance recommends that the high dose selected produce a pharmacodynamic response in dosed animals of such magnitude that further dose escalation would be precluded; it should not produce disturbances of physiology or homeostasis that would compromise the validity of the study.

Maximum Feasible Dose

ICH-2 also allows use of a MFD in the conduct of chronic rodent bioassays. The MFD by dietary administration is defined as 5% of the diet. When routes of administration other than dietary are appropriate, the high dose may be limited based on practical considerations and local tolerance.

SUMMARY

All countries and agencies examined in this chapter require high-dose testing in chronic animal bioassays as part of a protocol to assess the potential carcinogenicity of chemicals and other substances. Although terminology used to describe the highest dose differs to some extent between countries and agencies (e.g., MTD, minimally toxic dose, MFD, etc.), definitions of the highest dose seem to be remarkably similar among countries and organizations.

Most countries and organizations recognize the value of maximizing sensitivity of the bioassay at the highest dose and, to this end, require elicitation of some toxicity at the highest dose. The most common endpoints for assessment of toxicity are death and decrements in weight gain. However, many countries and organizations have begun to utilize other signs of toxicity such as tissue necrosis, metabolic saturation, organ-weight changes, hematology, urinalysis, clinical chemistry, pathology, histology, and toxicokinetics to determine the highest dose.

Factors that are used to select the middle and lowest doses include the relevance to human exposure as well as pharmacodynamic, toxicity, and mechanistic information. However, most countries and organizations do not use clearly articulated guidelines to select the middle and lowest doses for chronic rodent bioassays. Thus, the potential exists for significant international differences in the middle and lower doses selected for chronic bioassays because of a lack of guidelines for selection of these doses. However, these potential differences can be demonstrated only through direct examination of doses selected in several chemical-specific cases, a process that has not occurred to date.

REFERENCES

Barnes JM, Denz FA (1954) Experimental methods used in determining chronic toxicity: A critical review. Pharmacol Rev 6:191-242

Benitz KF (1970) Measurements of chronic toxicity. In Paget GE (ed), Methods in toxicology. Blackwell Scientific Publications, Oxford and Edinburgh, pp 82-131

Berenblum I, ed (1969) Carcinogenicity testing: a report of the Panel on Carcinogenicity of the Cancer Research Commission of the UICC. UICC Technical Report Series, vol 2

Chapin R, Bucher JR, Dieter M, et al (1994) National Toxicology Program (NTP) studies of glycol ethers. International Symposium on Health Hazards of Glycol Ethers, April 19–21, Nancy, France Clayson DB, Iverson F, Mueller R (1991) An appreciation of the maximum tolerated dose: an independently precise decision point in designing a carcinogenesis bioassay? Teratogenesis Carcinogenesis Mutagenesis 11:279–296

Clayson DB, Clegg DJ (1991) Classification of carcinogens: polemics, pedantics, or progress? Reg Toxicol Pharmacol 14: 147–166

Clayson DB (1962) Testing chemicals for carcinogenic activity, I: Methods. In Chemical carcinogenesis. J and A Churchill, Ltd, London, pp. 55-85

Commission of the European Communities (1980) Food-science and techniques. Reports of the Scientific Committee for Food, 10th series: Guidelines for the safety assessment of food additivcs

Commission of the European Communities (1989) Presentation of an application for assessment of a food additive prior to its approval. ECSC-EEC-EAEC Brussels. ISBN 92-826-0135-8

Commission of the European Communities (1990) Reports of the Scientific Committee for Food. Guidelines for the safety testing of food additives;

opinion expressed 22 February 1980. ISBN 92-825-2077-3

Committee on Carcinogenicity of Chemicals in Food, Consumer Products, and the Environment (1991) Guidelines for the evaluation of chemicals for carcinogenicity. Her Majesty's Stationery Office. ISBN 0-11-321453-7

Committee on Toxicity of Chemicals in Food, Consumer Products, and the Environment (CoT) (1982) Guidelines for the testing of chemicals for toxicity. Her majesty's Stationery Office. ISBN 0- 11-320815-4

Contrera JF, Jacobs A, Prassanna HR, et al (1995) A systemic exposure-based alternative to the maximum tolerated dose for carcinogenicity studies of human therapeutics. J Am College Toxicol 14:1–10

D'Aguanno W (1974) Drug safety evaluation: Pre-clinical considerations. In Fielding S, Lal H (eds), Neuroleptics. Futura Publishing Company, New York, pp 317-332

Della Porta G (1964) The study of chemical substances for possible carcinogenic actions. Proc Eur Soc Study Drug Toxicity 3:29-40

Department of Health and Social Security, Committee on Carcinogenicity of Chemicals in Food (1979) Consumer products and the environment: a consultative document on guidelines for the testing of chemicals for carcinogenicity. Her Majesty's Stationery Office, London

European Communities—67/548/EEC (1967) Council Directive of 27 June 1967 on the approximation of laws, regulations and administrative provisions relating to the classification, packaging, and labeling of dangerous substances. Official J Eur Communities Special Ed, No L 154/1 35:234–237

European Communities—91/414/EEC (1991) Council Directive of 15 July 1991 concerning the placing of plant protection products on the market. Official J Eur Communities Legislation, No L 230/1 34

European Communities—92/32/EEC (1992) Council Directive of 30 April 1992 amending for the seventh time Directive 67/538/EEC on the approximation of the laws, regulations, and administrative provisions relating to the classification, packaging and labeling of dangerous substances. Official J Eur Communities Legislation No L 154/1 35

Fitzhugh OG (1955) VI Chronic oral toxicity. Food Drug Cosmet Law J, pp 712-719

Food and Drug Administration, Advisory Committee on Protocols for Safety Evaluation (1971). Panel on Carcinogenesis report on cancer testing in the safety evaluation of food additives and pesticides. Toxicol Appl Pharmacol 20:419-438

Food Safety Council (1980) Proposed systems for food safety assessment. FSC, Washington, DC

Friedman L (1974) Section 4: Report of Discussion Group No. 3: Dose selection and administration. In Golberg L (ed), Carcinogenesis testing of chemicals. CRC Press, Cleveland, pp 21-22

Grice HC (ed) (1984) The selection of doses in chronic toxicity/carcinogenecity studies. Springer-Verlag, New York

Haseman JK, Lockhart A (1994) The relationship between use of the maximum tolerated dose and study sensitivity for detecting rodent carcinogenicity.

Fundam Appl Toxicol 22:382–394
Hayashi Y (1992) Overview of genotoxic carcinogens and non- genotoxic carcinogens. Exp Toxicol Pathol 44:465–472
Health and Welfare Canada (1975) The testing of chemicals for carcinogenicity, mutagenicity, and teratogenicity. Health and Welfare Canada, Ottawa, pp 2-31
Health Canada (1991) Carcinogen Assessment. Health Protection Branch
Huff J, Bucher JR, Schwetz BA, Barrett JC (1994) Optimum exposure levels for chemical carcinogenesis experiments: concepts, principles, guidelines, and experience. Abstract 475 presented at the 1994 Annual Meeting of the Society of Toxicology, Dallas, TX ICH-1 Recommendations on Carcinogenicity Testing (1992) In D'Arcy PF, Harron WDG (eds) Proceedings of First International Conference on Harmonization, Brussels, 1991. Greystone Books, Northern Ireland, pp 185–186
Interagency Regulatory Liaison Group, Work Group on Risk Assessment (1979) Scientific bases for identification of potential. J NatlCancer Inst 63:241-268
Interagency Staff Group on Carcinogens, U.S. (1986) Chemical carcinogens: A review of the science and its associated principles. Environ Health Perspec 67:201–282
International Agency for Research on Cancer (1980) Long-term and short-term screening assays for carcinogens: a critical appraisal. IARC Monographs on the Evaluation of the Carcinogenic Risk of Chemicals to Humans, Supplement 2. International Agency for Research on Cancer, Lyons, France
International Agency for Research on Cancer (1980) Long-term and short-term screening assays for carcinogenesis: a critical appraisal. Supplement 2. IARC, Lyons, France
International Conference on Harmonisation of Technical Requirements for Registration of Pharmaceuticals for Human Use (1995) Fed Register 60:11278 (March 1995)
Loomis TA (1968) Essentials of toxicology. Lea and Febiger, Philadelphia, pp 139-156
Magee PN (1970) Tests for carcinogenic potential. In Paget GE (ed), Methods in toxicology. Blackwell Scientific Publications, Oxford and Edinburgh, pp 158-196
McConnell EE (1989) The maximum tolerated dose: the debate. J Am College Toxicol 8:115–1112
Ministry of Agriculture, Forestry and Fisheries (1985) Guidance on toxicology study data for application of agriculture chemical registration. Notification of Agricultural Production Bureau, 59 Nosan No. 4200, January 28
Ministry of Health and Welfare, Japan (1984) Guidelines for toxicity studies of drugs. Notification No. 118 of the Pharmaceutical Affairs Bureau, February 15
Ministry of Health and Welfare, Japan (1988) Guidelines for toxicity studies of new animal drugs. Notification No. 63-44 of the Drug Bureau, March 31
Ministry of Health and Welfare, Japan (1989) Guidelines for toxicity studies

of drugs. Notification No. 24 of First and Second Evaluation and Registration Divisions, and Biologics and Antibiotics Division, September 11

Ministry of Health and Welfare, Japan (1990) Guideline for toxicity testing of chemicals. In Environmental Health Bureau (ed), Guide Book on New Chemical Substance Registration. Yakugyo- Jiho-Sha, Tokyo, pp 219–238

Ministry of Health and Welfare, Japan (1993) Guidelines for toxicity studies of drugs. Notification No. 88 of New Drugs Division, August 10

National Research Council (1977) Drinking Water and Health. National Academy Press, Washington, DC

National Research Council (1993) Use of the maximum tolerated dose in animal bioassays for carcinogenicity. In Goldstein B, et al (eds), Issues in Risk Assessment. National Academy Press, Washington, DC, pp 15–83

National Toxicology Program Board of Scientific Counselors (1984) Report of the NTP Ad Hoc Panel on Chemical Carcinogenesis Testing and Evaluation. U.S. Department of Health and Human Services, Public Health Service, National Institutes of Health, Bethesda, MD (August 17)

National Toxicology Program Board of Scientific Counselors (1992) Final Report of the Advisory Review. Fed Register 57:31721–31730 (July 17)

National Toxicology Program (1993a) NTP Technical Report on the Toxicity and Carcinogenicity of Oxazepam in Swiss-Webster and B6C3F1 Mice. NIH Publication 92-3359. U.S. Department of Health and Human Services, Public Health Service, National Institutes of Health, Bethesda, MD

National Toxicology Program (1993b) NTP Technical Report on Toxicology and Carcinogenesis Studies of 1,3-Butadiene in B6C3F1 Mice. NIH Publication 93-3165. U.S. Department of Health and Human Services, Public Health Service, National Institutes of Health, Bethesda, MD

National Toxicology Program (1993c) Toxicology and Carcinogenesis Studies of Polybrominated Biphenyls in F344/N Rats and B6C3F1 Mice. NIH Publication 93-2853. U.S. Department of Health and Human Services, Public Health Service, National Institutes of Health, Bethesda, MD

Newberne PM (1975) Pathology: Studies of chronic toxicity and carcinogenicity. J Assoc Off Anal Chem 58:650-656

Office of Science and Technology Policy (1985) Chemical carcinogens: A review of the science and its associated principles. Fed Register Part II:10371–10442 (March 14) Sontag JR, Page NP, Safiotti U (1976) Guidelines for Carcinogen Bioassay in Small Rodents. NIH Publication 76-801. National Cancer Institute, Bethesda, MD

Organization of Economic and Cooperative Development, Long-Term Expert Group (1981) Test guidelines for carcinogenicity studies

Page NP (1977a) Chronic toxicity and carcinogenicity guidelines. J Environ Pathol Toxicol 1:161-182

Page NP (1977b) Concepts of a bioassay program in environmental carcinogenesis. In Kraybill HF, Mehlman MA (eds), Environmental cancer. Advances in Modern Toxicology, vol 3. Hemisphere, Washington, pp 108-113

Peck HM (1974) Design of experiments to detect carcinogenic effects of drugs. In Golberg L (ed), Carcinogenic testing of chemicals. CRC Press, Cleveland, pp 1-13

Sontag JM, Page NP, Saffiotti U (1976) Guidelines for carcinogen bioassay in small rodents. National Institutes of Health, DHEW Publication No (NIH) 76-801. National Institutes of Health, Bethesda, MD

Travlos GS, Morris RW, Elwell MR, et al (1996) Frequency and relationships of clinical chemistry and liver and kidney histopathology findings in 13-week toxicity studies in rats. Toxicology 107:17–29

U.S. Environmental Protection Agency (1986) Guidelines for Carcinogenic Risk Assessment. Fed Register 51:33992–34003

U.S. Environmental Protection Agency (1987) Position Paper on the Selection of a Maximum Tolerated Dose (MTD) on Carcinogenicity Studies. National Technical Information Service, Springfield, VA

U.S. Environmental Protection Agency (1989) Health Effects Test Guidelines, Office of Toxic Substances. Fed Register 54:21064

Weisburger JH, Weisburger EK (1967) Tests for chemical carcinogenesis. In Busch H, Methods in cancer research, vol 1. Academic Press, New York, pp 307-398

World Health Organization (1969) Principles for the testing and evaluation of drugs for carcinogenicity: report of a WHO scientific group. World Health Organization Technical Report Series, No 426. WHO, Geneva

World Health Organization (1978). Principles and methods for evaluating toxicity of chemicals, Part 1. Environmental Health Criteria, vol. 6. WHO, Geneva

Chapter 3

Implications of International Differences in Dose Selection[1]

INTRODUCTION

International differences in dose selection regimens for chronic rodent bioassays may have an impact on issues other than the interpretation of the assay results. Results of rodent bioassays for carcinogenicity and systemic toxicity are used by national governments to approve the introduction into commerce of industrial chemicals and pesticides and to approve the import and export of industrial chemicals and pesticides or products containing chemicals or pesticides.

It is not unusual for companies to test a chemical for carcinogenicity or systemic toxicity in one country and submit the results to another country with the intent of receiving marketing approval (for either the raw chemical or its formulated products) in that country. When testing requirements (i.e., for dose selection) differ between countries, data from a bioassay conducted for one country and submitted to another for regulatory considerations may be rejected. In this case, the company either may be required to conduct a new bioassay on the chemical or may choose not to market the chemical or its formulated products in the second country.

In this chapter, we examine the acceptance or rejection of data from chronic rodent bioassays in several countries based on dose selection procedures. This analysis is drawn from the 1993 study of pesticide registration rejections by the United States Environmental Protection Agency, Office of Pesticide Programs (EPA 1993). As described in Chapter 2, the EPA requires the highest dose in a chronic rodent bioassay to meet their definition of a maximum tolerated dose (MTD). Although many other countries require use of a MTD, they may define the term differently or, more likely, interpret achievement of the highest dose (and related phenomena such as overdose) differently. The results of these differences are demonstrated in the following case studies for selected pesticides. This analysis does not address nonpesticidal chemicals; therefore, the results may not be applicable to other types of industrial chemicals. Further, some of these bioassays and associated decisions were conducted and made several years ago; as such, the decisions may not reflect current regulatory philosophy, particularly in the United States.

---

[1] Contributions to this chapter were made by M. vanGemert, J. T. Stevens, R. A. Cardona, and S. Hurt.

REGISTRATION REJECTION RATE: ENVIRONMENTAL PROTECTION AGENCY

Achievement of the MTD was a critical factor in the acceptance or rejection of rodent bioassays for pesticide registration in the United States (EPA 1993). Fifty-one of 149 mouse studies (34%) and 58 of 172 bioassays (33%) were rejected or declared supplemental primarily because the MTD was not achieved (EPA 1993). The results of this analysis are depicted in Figure 1 by year of EPA review.

During the review period 1986–1988, when the EPA issued the Maximum Tolerated Dose Position Document of 1987 (Farber 1987), the document did not appear to have a significant impact on the rate of mouse bioassay rejection. However, the rate of rat bioassay rejection increased during this period. Further, an improved acceptance rate during the post-1988 period was noted for both rat and mouse bioassays (Figure 1). It is assumed that the improved acceptance rate occurred as industry adjusted to the new standard.

An update of these data suggests that the true rejection rate (i.e., not including those studies that were declared supplemental) was approximately 12% for the rat and 5% for the mouse. Between 1993 and 1995, no cancer studies conducted for reregistration were rejected outright (Caulkins, per-

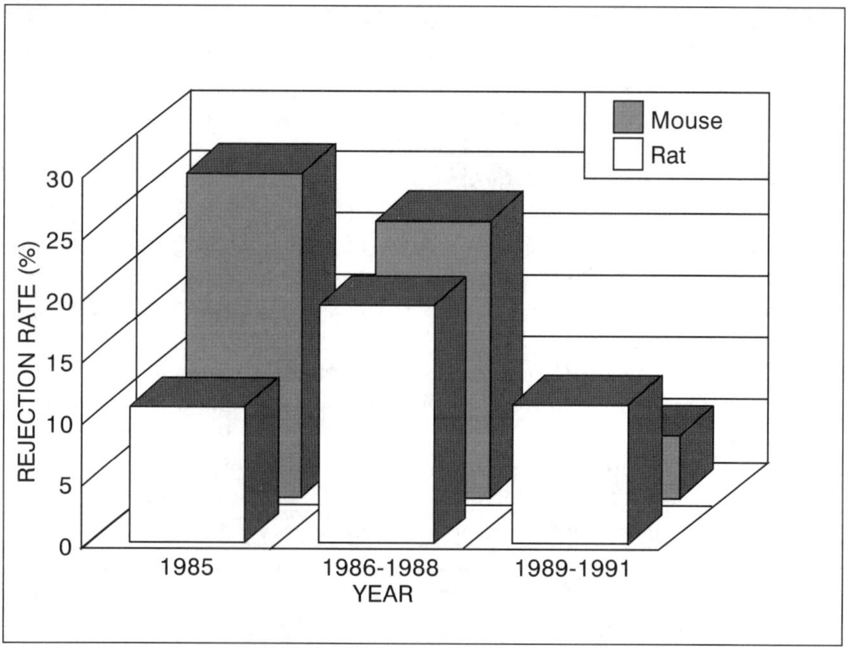

Figure 1. The EPA rejection rate analysis.

sonal communication). Further, it should be noted that the EPA does not necessarily ask that all studies that are rejected or declared supplemental be repeated. In fact, in many cases, additional clarification of the existing data or generation of new data in a short-term study (28–90 days) is sufficient to resolve the EPA's concern and allow (re)registration activity to go forward.

At the joint Guideline Harmonization Workshop held in Washington, DC, in October 1992, the Organization for Economic Cooperation and Development (OECD) indicated that the EPA's reliance on the MTD may represent a major barrier to harmonization of testing methodologies and, ultimately, free trade. To address this issue, the OECD requested that examples be provided where the highest dose in a rodent bioassay was perceived to be too low or adequate by the EPA but adequate or too high by other countries. The following limited sampling of case studies, representing a study population approaching 100, presents the results of the analysis of data submitted to fulfill the OECD request. Accompanying this analysis are the regulatory decisions that were made by various countries based on the data submitted for registration purposes.

CASE STUDIES

The case studies presented here represent two types of analyses and regulatory decisions influenced by high-dose selection. First, examples of cases when the EPA concluded that the highest dose tested was too low (did not achieve the MTD), whereas other countries accepted the highest dose tested (2,4-D, dimethipin, myclobutanil, and penconazole) are discussed. In some of these cases the EPA approved the pesticide registration and in some cases rejected it. Second, cases when the highest dose tested met the EPA requirement for the MTD but exceeded high-dose requirements in other countries (acetate, propiconazole, and 1,1-dimethylhydrazine [UDMH]) are discussed. A final case study is provided for the herbicide primisulfuron-methyl, which was registered in the United States based on data where the MTD was clearly exceeded. In this case, toxicokinetic data were used to demonstrate that the highest doses exceeded a metabolic breakpoint.

Case 1: Highest Dose Too Low (United States)/Adequate (non-United States)

2,4-D

Chronic toxicity/carcinogenicity studies in Fischer 344 rats and B6C3Fl mice were submitted to the EPA in 1986. Comparable doses were selected for both studies—0, 1, 15, and 45 mg per kg of body weight. The EPA reviewed these studies upon receipt and presented the reviews to the EPA Cancer Peer

Review Committee, which called both studies supplementary, stating that, although these studies were adequate in design, a MTD had not been achieved. Signs of toxicity in the mouse included histologic changes in the renal tubular epithelium in males at 15 mg/kg and 45 mg/kg and increased kidney weights in both males and females at 45 mg/kg. In the rat study, signs of toxicity included increased brown tubular cell pigment in males and females at 5 mg/kg, increased pelvic microcalculi in males at 15 mg/kg and in males and females at 45 mg/kg, and increased transitional epithelial hyperplasia in females at 45 mg/kg.

On June 25, 1987, the Federal Insecticide, Fungicide, and Rodenticide Act (FIFRA) Scientific Advisory Panel (SAP) reviewed the two studies and concluded that: 1) the 2,4-D rat and mouse carcinogenicity studies were adequate in design and conduct; 2) the data were negative for carcinogenicity in female rats and both sexes of mice; and 3) they did not agree with the EPA Cancer Peer Review Committee's conclusion that the compound should be classified as an interim C (possible human carcinogen). The SAP stated that an increased incidence of astrocytomas in male rats exposed to 2,4-D at 45 mg/kg was equivocal evidence of carcinogenicity. Therefore, registrants should conduct an additional rat study to address astrocytomas only, with two male control groups of 50 animals each and two male test groups of the same size exposed to 2,4-D at 45 mg/kg.

The EPA did not follow the recommendations of the SAP. A July 1989 notice from the EPA (special data call-in for 2,4-D) required standard oral exposure testing of male and female rats and mice with technical-grade 2,4-D because the EPA determined that the MTD was not reached in any chronic or subchronic studies. The registrants also were required to perform the necessary subchronic toxicity tests to determine and support appropriate dose levels for the carcinogenicity tests. These actions were required despite the fact that the original bioassays were accepted as a portion of the database for the registration of 2,4-D in 28 other countries.

Dimethipin (Harvade)

The study in question was a chronic/carcinogenicity study using Sprague–Dawley CD rats with dietary doses of 0, 40, 200, or 1000 ppm. Originally, the EPA accepted this study. However, the EPA Cancer Peer Review Committee reviewed the study on January 5, 1990, and stated that it should be repeated for the reregistration process. This decision was influenced by results of a carcinogenicity study conducted in CD-1 mice. Dimethipin produced a slightly elevated incidence of pulmonary adenomas/carcinomas combined in male (but not female) mice at the highest dose tested.

At the Peer Review Committee's deliberations on the results of the rat study, members noted the absence of significant toxicity at the highest dose, the presence of decreased body weight gains of 7–13%, the existence of increased liver weights, and evidence of focally dilated bile ducts (which did not appear to be life-threatening). They further stated that in the 90-day subchronic study, the highest dose (1000 ppm) was a no-effect level. On this basis, the committee concluded that a MTD had not been achieved in the rat study and that it should be repeated.

Dimethipin has been registered in 18 countries as a result of the original rat study. This study also was reviewed and accepted by the Joint Meeting on Pesticide Residues (JMPR) panel of the World Health Organization (WHO) in 1985 and 1988, and the highest dose tested in this study was not considered an issue by the Food and Agriculture Organization (FAO)/WHO (1985, 1988).

Myclobutanil

The EPA accepted both the rat and mouse chronic/ carcinogenicity studies as the basis for a conditional registration granted in 1989, as no evidence of carcinogenic potential was found in either of these studies. However, the EPA required that new carcinogenicity studies be conducted as a condition for registration, because the agency concluded that a MTD had not been reached in male and female rats or in female mice.

In the rat study, Sprague–Dawley rats were exposed to 0, 50, 200, or 800 ppm. The effects observed were decreased testicular weight and increased testicular atrophy at the middle dose, with decreased body weight gain and food consumption, increased liver weight, decreased testicular weight, and increased testicular atrophy at the highest dose tested. The EPA concluded that the MTD approximated 3000 ppm based on a 13–17% decrease in body weight gain at this level in the 90-day study.

In the mouse study, CD-1 mice were exposed to 0, 20, 100, or 500 ppm for 24 months. At the middle dose, hepatic mixed function oxidase activity increased at 3, 6, and 12 months in males and females. At the high dose, the liver showed increased foci of altered cells, increased hepatocellular vacuolation, and increased liver weights in both males and females. No effects on body weight, food consumption, or survival were found. However, body-weight gain was decreased 10–15% during the first 90 days of the study. The EPA concluded that 1000 ppm in males and 3000 ppm in females in the 90-day study exceeded the MTD because of 35% and 37% decreases in body weight gain, respectively, at these levels and concluded that the females had not been adequately challenged.

These original rat and mouse studies have been accepted in support of new product registrations in more than 40 countries. In addition, no high-dose issues were raised in the review of myclobutanil by the 1992 WHO JMPR panel, as they concurred that myclobutanil was not carcinogenic in rats or mice (FAO/WHO 1993a).

(Note: The registrant elected to conduct the required studies, and the findings in the new higher-dose studies were consistent with those observed in the earlier studies, reflecting dose-related severity with no evidence of carcinogenic potential. The absence of a decrease in survival confirmed the EPA's position *that higher doses could have been fed in the original studies.)*

Penconazole (Registration Rejected in the United States)

Two chronic/carcinogenicity studies in RAIf Sprague–Dawley rats and TIF mice were submitted to the EPA in 1988. In the rat study, 80 animals/sex/group were dosed with 0, 0.25, 3.75, 7.5, or 15 mg/kg with effects of increased liver weights at the interim and terminal sacrifice found at 7.5 and 15 mg/kg. In the mouse study, doses of 0, 0.7, 10.7, 21.4, or 42.8 mg/kg were fed in the diet. Effects on adrenal weights were observed at the 21.4-mg/kg dose. At 42.8 mg/kg, increases in liver weights were seen at interim sacrifice. The dose rates for both studies were clearly supported based on the subchronic studies conducted with penconazole. However, the EPA declared these studies inadequate because the MTD had not been achieved. As a result, the registrant withdrew the petition for registration of this product (EPA 1989).

The WHO accepted these same studies in 1992 and published its findings in 1993 (FAO/WHO 1993b); over 40 other countries have accepted these studies without considering the top dose inadequate.

Case 2: Highest Dose Met Requirements (United States)/ Exceeded Requirements (non-United States)

Acephate

A carcinogenicity study was conducted with acephate in which Charles River CD-1 mice (75/sex/dose) were fed diets containing 0, 50, 250, or 1000 ppm of acephate for 24 months. An increase in the incidence of hepatocellular carcinoma, apparently unrelated to liver toxicity, was observed in female mice receiving 1000 ppm. The authors concluded that the MTD had been exceeded on the basis of a marked decrease in body weight (24% for males and 25% for females). In addition, liver and lung histopathologic changes were seen at the high dose. At the middle dose (250 ppm), toxicity was observed that included decreased body weight (11% in males and 14% in females) and liver and lung histopathologic changes.

The EPA reviewed and accepted these studies for registration purposes, although the FIFRA SAP concluded that the MTD was exceeded on the basis of body weight but not survival. The panel went on to say that acephate could be categorized in either carcinogen group C or D. The presence of positive genotoxic data was considered pivotal in placing acephate in group C.

The FAO/WHO JMPR panel reviewed the mouse carcinogenicity study with acephate in 1987 (FAO/WHO 1987a) and concluded: "The liver changes observed in this study occurred in a dose-related manner and were maximal at doses that were clearly toxic. An increase in liver to body-weight ratio also occurred that was statistically significant in high-dose females. Hepatocyte hypertrophy in response to enzyme induction with subsequent hyperplasia, adenoma formation, and in some instances, to carcinoma, is not remarkable and is of doubtful prognostic significance for man."

Acephate has been registered for use on food crops in over 55 countries with no concern about a tumor response at the highest dose tested. In the majority of these countries, this tumor response is looked at as an overdose phenomenon associated with a nongenotoxic chemical.

Propiconazole

Propiconazole was found not to be mutagenic in 22 independent studies, not teratogenic, and not carcinogenic in Sprague–Dawley rats or female CD-1 mice (at levels exceeding the MTD) (Stevens et al. 1992). However, an increase in liver tumors was observed in male CD-1 mice at the MTD.

A combined toxicity/carcinogenicity study was performed in CD-1 mice at dose levels of 0, 100, 500, and 2500 ppm and was submitted to and accepted by the EPA in 1989. An increase in benign and malignant liver tumors was seen in male mice at feeding levels that appeared to exceed the MTD. At the high dose, a 30–40% reduction in body-weight gain was observed, as was a significant reduction in survival in males during the first year of the study. An increase in SGOT and SGPT was observed and the incidence of liver tumors was significantly higher than the spontaneous rate in male mice. Liver weights at the high dose were increased in both sexes.

At the middle dose, the toxicologic findings included a significant reduction in body-weight gain in the first year in males, accompanied by changes in hypertrophy of the hepatocytes as well as an elevation in SGOT. No increase in tumors was seen at the 12-month interim kill.

The EPA's Cancer Peer Review Committee met and issued a memo in April 1987 classifying propiconazole as a category C (possible human carcinogen). However, the FIFRA SAP classified propiconazole as a category D carcinogen and stated that mathematical risk assessment should not be used in estimating risk.

Propiconazole has been registered in 75 countries for use on cereal and fruit crops. It was registered first in France in 1980. It has no restrictions as a potential carcinogen as most countries treat the response observed in male mice fed 2500 ppm in their diet for 2 years as an overdose phenomenon. The FAO/WHO JMPR panel accepted the study in 1987 with no classification of the chemical as a carcinogen (FAO/WHO 1987b).

UDMH

Two CD-1 mouse carcinogenicity studies were conducted with UDMH (1,1-dimethylhydrazine), a by-product and impurity in daminozide, and submitted to the EPA. One study was performed at doses of 0, 1, 5, 10, and 20 ppm; the other was performed at doses of 0, 40, and 80 ppm. Increases in hemangiomas and hemangiosarcomas were found at 40 and 80 ppm but not at lower doses. The increased tumor incidence was accompanied by excessive mortality and clinical pathology indicative of hepatotoxicity and toxicity to the hematopoietic system. The extent of toxicity observed provided evidence that the MTD was exceeded. However, the EPA evaluated the study and accepted the results at the higher doses, concluding that the highest dose was adequate for carcinogenicity testing in males, although females may have tolerated higher doses.

The EPA's Cancer Peer Review Committee concluded that there was significant liver toxicity, especially in male mice, which did not appear to be life-threatening. They concluded that the high rate of mortality observed in the second year of the high-dose study appeared to be the result of neoplasms and not excessive dosing. Also, the types of liver tumors seen in the study (hemangiomas and hemangiosarcomas) are not considered relevant to the type of hepatocellular toxicity observed, especially when the type of liver necrosis observed appeared to be limited to single-cell necrosis.

The FAO/WHO JMPR panel rejected the high-dose study in 1991, indicating that the high mortality and severe toxicity observed in animals treated with 40 and 80 ppm confounded interpretation and suggested that the MTD was exceeded. The United Kingdom partially accepted the studies in 1989 and concluded that the MTD may have been exceeded (Ministry of Agriculture, Fisheries and Food 1989).

Although an acceptable daily intake of 0.5 mg per kg of body weight was established by the WHO in 1989 for daminozide containing the by-product UDMH, worldwide registration for daminozide on food crops was withdrawn by the manufacturer because of the EPA's conclusions about the significance of the high-dose CD-1 mouse study.

Case 3: Highest Dose Exceeded: Influence of Toxicokinetic Data

Primisulfuron-methyl

Primisulfuron-methyl is a sulfonylurea herbicide. Its structure is shown in Figure 2.

Primisulfuron-methyl is not highly acutely toxic and is not a potential sensitizing agent; nor is it mutagenic, teratogenic, a reproductive toxin, or carci-

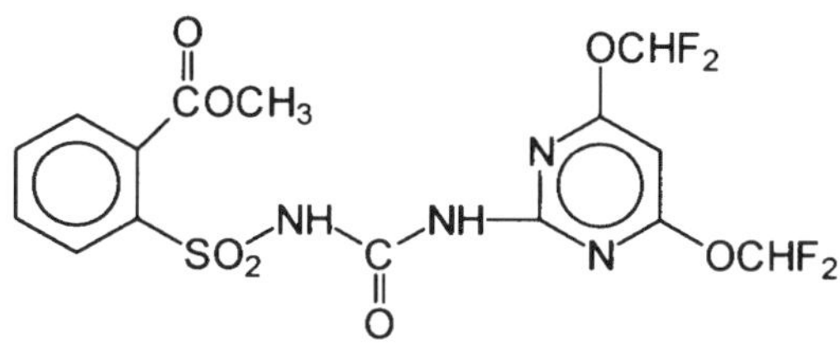

Figure 2. Primisulfuron-methyl.

nogenic in rats. At feeding levels greater than 3000 ppm in male mice and 10,000 ppm in female mice, hepatocellular tumors were observed. However, at these levels of primisulfuron-methyl administration the MTD was clearly exceeded, as evidenced by marked effects on body weight, body-weight gain, liver toxicity, fluorosis, and, most importantly, reduced survival. On the basis of these effects, the EPA and its SAP concluded with the sponsor that primisulfuron-methyl is not classifiable for carcinogenicity (category D).

Toxicokinetic studies evaluating the fecal metabolite profile after dietary administration of primisulfuron-methyl at 100, 500, 1000, 5000, 10,000, and 20,000 ppm revealed the appearance of a new metabolite in male and female mice at feeding levels of 5000 ppm. The structure of the unique fecal metabolite occurring at feeding levels of 5000 ppm and above is presented in Figure 3 (Stevens and Sumner 1991, 1994).

This high feeding level metabolite is a dimer of the original compound with a ring difluoromethyl group replaced with a disulfide bridge. The high molecular weight of this dimer suggests that this product is secreted into the bile from the liver. The difluoromethoxy groups remain intact in other metabolites isolated from mice and rats, which suggests that the pathway is unique at

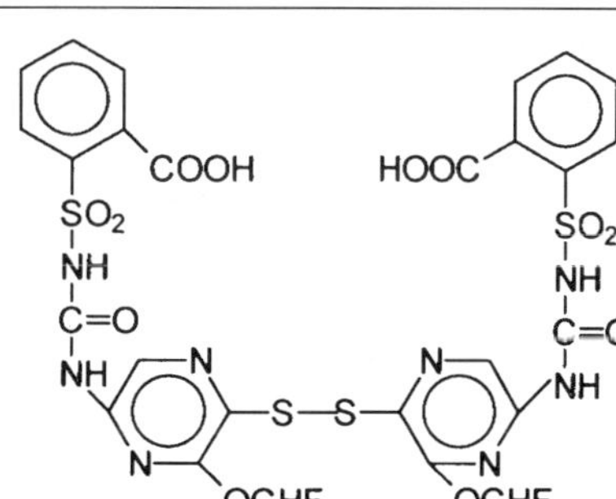

Figure 3. Fecal metabolite dimer.

these high doses. The loss of the difluoromethoxy groups, freeing up fluorine, might explain the fluorosis, which is evident only at high feeding levels.

An additional carcinogenicity study was completed with primisulfuron-methyl in male and female CD-1 mice fed doses of 0, 500, 1000, or 1500 ppm in the diet. In this study, the MTD was considered to be near 1500 ppm based on evidence of liver centrilobular hypertrophy, nephropathy, and testicular degeneration. However, there was no increase in neoplastic lesions of any type or in any organ, including the liver, for those mice fed primisulfuron-methyl in their diet at levels up to and including 1500 ppm. The liver tumor response and fluorosis in mice observed at feeding levels in excess of the MTD can be attributed to a metabolic overload. This overload was identified by a qualitative alteration in the metabolite production, which does not occur with the dietary administration of primisulfuron-methyl at or below the MTD.

Primisulfuron-methyl has been registered in 11 countries besides the United States since its introduction in 1990. In no instance has there been concern about the tumor response in mice. These 11 countries, like the United States, consider the response observed with primisulfuron-methyl to be an overdose phenomenon and the results at the highest doses not to be relevant to human health risk assessment.

CONCLUSIONS

The information presented in this analysis indicates that reliance on different definitions of the highest dose in chronic rodent studies has led to differences in the acceptance or rejection of data submitted for regulatory purposes in different countries throughout the world. Because of these differences, the potential exists for conflicting regulatory decisions on chemicals or products containing those chemicals and, ultimately, for rejection of import tolerances with resultant barriers to trade.

The worth of agricultural food production that is traded annually on a worldwide basis is substantial and, with the expectation that the level of food trade will grow to more than $300 billion by the year 2000, reduction of the potential for trade barriers seems prudent, particularly where trade is constrained without commensurate improvements in protection of human health. International harmonization of dose-selection procedures seems a worthy effort where it can reduce conflicting regulatory decisions, reduce the potential for restriction of trade for critical food and other products, and adequately protect public health.

REFERENCES

Farber T (1987) United States Environmental Protection Agency. Pesticide Assessment Guidelines, Subdivision F, Position Document—Selection of a Maximum Tolerated Dose (MTD) in Oncogenicity Studies. National Technical Information Service, Washington, DC

Food and Agriculture Organization/World Health Organization (1985) Report of the Joint Meeting of the FAO Panel of Expert Group on Pesticide Residues in Food and the WHO Expert Group on Pesticide Residues. Pesticide Residues in Food—1985. FAO Plant Protection Paper. FAO/WHO, Geneva, pp 55–73

Food and Agriculture Organization/World Health Organization (1987a) Report of the Joint Meeting of the FAO Panel of Expert Group on Pesticide Residues in Food and the WHO Expert Group on Pesticide Residues. Pesticide Residues in Food—1987. FAO Plant Protection Paper. FAO/WHO, Rome, pp 68–73

Food and Agriculture Organization/World Health Organization (1987b) Report of the Joint Meeting of the FAO Panel of Expert Group on Pesticide Residues in Food and the WHO Expert Group on Pesticide Residues. Pesticide Residues in Food—1987. FAO Plant Protection Paper. FAO/WHO, Rome, pp 62–67

Food and Agriculture Organization/World Health Organization (1988) Report of the Joint Meeting of the FAO Panel of Expert Group on Pesticide Residues in Food and the WHO Expert Group on Pesticide Residues. Pesticide Residues in Food—1988. FAO Plant Protection Paper. FAO/WHO, Rome, pp 19–21

Food and Agriculture Organization/World Health Organization (1993a) Report of the Joint Meeting of the FAO Panel of Expert Group on Pesticide Residues in Food and the WHO Expert Group on Pesticide Residues. Pesticide Residues in Food—1992. FAO Plant Protection Paper 116. FAO/WHO, Rome, pp 62–66

Food and Agriculture Organization/World Health Organization (1993b) Report of the Joint Meeting of the FAO Panel of Expert Group on Pesticide Residues in Food and the WHO Expert Group on Pesticide Residues. Pesticide Residues in Food—1992. FAO Plant Protection Paper 116. FAO/WHO, Rome, pp 71–74

Ministry of Agriculture, Fisheries and Food: Advisory Committee on Pesticides (1989) Position Document on Consumer Risk Arising from the Use of Products containing Daminozole on Apples and Pears

Stevens JT, Barnett JW, Breckenridge CB, Thompson SS (1992) Safety Evaluation of Propiconazole. Toxicologist 12(10):112

Stevens JT, Sumner DD (1991) The value of biokinetic data in hazard and risk assessment. In Rescigno A, Thakur AK (eds), New Trends In Pharmacokinetics, Plenum, New York, pp 315–333

Stevens JT, Sumner DD (1994) Pharmacokinetic factors influencing risk assessment: Saturation of absorption and active transport; dose-dependent metabolite production; and co-factor depletion. Environ Health Perspect 102(Suppl. 11):13–22

U.S. Environmental Protection Agency (1989) Withdrawn Petition. PP 8F3657. Fed Register 54(192):41160–41161

U.S. Environmental Protection Agency (1993) Pesticide Reregistration Rejection Rate Analysis: Toxicology. EPA 738-R-93-004. pp 50–54

Chapter 4

Factors Influencing Dose Selection[1]

INTRODUCTION

The selection of the highest, middle, and lowest doses in a chronic rodent bioassay is influenced by two critical factors: study objective and practical (biological/chemical) considerations. This chapter examines these factors as they influence dose selection for bioassays of environmental chemicals. Although the focus of this chapter, as well as the entire monograph, is on dose selection for bioassays of environmental chemicals, some of the factors that influence dose selection for pharmaceuticals (Weissinger 1992, Davies 1992, Usui 1992, International Conference on Harmonisation 1995) appear relevant for environmental chemicals and also are discussed.

SELECTION OF THE HIGHEST DOSE

Chronic rodent bioassays typically are conducted to evaluate the potential hazard of a compound, to assess the dose-response relationship, to make determinations of safety, or a combination of these objectives. The highest dose for chronic rodent bioassays may differ depending upon the study objective, and objectives are discussed in this chapter in the context of the framework for human health risk assessment (National Research Council 1983).

Dose Selection Based on Study Objective

Hazard Identification

Hazard identification is the step in a formal risk assessment where the potential adverse effects of human exposure to a substance are identified. The step includes an assessment of the potential for the substance to elicit an array of effects in humans including carcinogenicity, reproductive and developmental toxicity, neurotoxicity, and others. Most information on potential hazard is provided by animal and human epidemiologic studies, with some information derived from in vitro assays. Dose selection is addressed in this monograph only in the context of animal studies (chronic rodent assays).

---

[1]Contributions to this chapter were made by the ILSI Risk Science Institute Working Group on Dose Selection for Chronic Rodent Bioassays.

One goal for chronic rodent bioassays of potential carcinogens in the context of hazard identification is to reduce the likelihood of a false-negative result. It has been suggested that, with typical bioassays of 50 animals per dose, an excess tumor incidence of at least 10% is required for the effect to be statistically detectable (Haseman 1985). However, the excess tumor incidence necessary to provide a statistically measurable response will be dependent on the background incidence and tumor type. Haseman (1985) has suggested that a reasonably high probability (90%) of detecting an increase for a tumor with a spontaneous incidence rate of 0.1% requires a dose high enough to elicit a tumor incidence of 15.8%. For a common tumor with a background rate of 20% or higher, the dose would have to be high enough to produce a tumor rate of 56% for a 90% chance of detection (Haseman 1985). Consequently, the 50-animal bioassay is unable to detect relatively weak carcinogens at any dose and relatively potent carcinogens at low doses.

Selection of the highest dose also is constrained by toxicity in test organisms; that is, the highest dose is selected so as not to cause overt toxicity other than toxicity associated with the effect of interest (e.g., carcinogenicity). As discussed in Chapter 2, the definition of overt toxicity differs between countries and regulatory agencies, although all countries and agencies utilize at least one relatively high dose, presumably to maximize study sensitivity.

The sensitivity of current animal bioassays conducted with the maximum tolerated dose (MTD) is sufficiently high that nearly all known human carcinogens also are positive animal carcinogens (Huff and Rall 1992), although target organ concordance is much lower than the sensitivity of the assay and it is not always known whether the mechanism of tumor formation is the same in both species. However, specificity with respect to the production of false-negative results is more difficult to address because of a paucity of, or weaknesses in, epidemiologic studies for most chemicals.

Questions of high-dose testing have been raised associated with the potential for disease (primarily cancer) induced by mechanisms that are not operative at lower doses in either humans or test animals. Higher doses also may induce tumors that kill the test animals before sufficient time has passed to allow expression of other tumors that might be observed at lower doses. When a high dose elicits disease by a mechanism not operative at lower doses, or in humans exposed to considerably lower doses, the relevance of a positive assay at a high dose to human risk may be questioned. Mechanisms that may be operative only, or to a disproportionate degree, at high doses in chronic rodent bioassays include induced cell proliferation, saturation of metabolic capacity, hormonal imbalance, or other biochemical or physiologic changes. When it is suspected that such mechanisms are operative in the carcinogenic process, it is important to determine that these mechanisms are inoperative in humans at environmentally relevant exposures.

Selection of doses for substances that act by what may be unique mechanisms at high doses is problematic. The NRC Committee on Risk Assessment Methodologies (NRC 1993) recommended to continue the use of a high dose defined as the MTD and, when assays are positive, to gather additional data to address human relevance after the fact. However, a minority of the NRC committee suggested that the highest dose should be selected that will yield relevant data to predict human risk, relying on information from subchronic studies that elucidates the mechanism of action, effects on biochemical and physiologic processes, effects on cell proliferation and hormonal imbalance, etc.

Dose-Response Assessment

Dose-response assessment is an inherently quantitative step in the formal risk assessment process and involves articulation of the potency of the compound as defined by the shape and slope of the dose-response curve. Goals of this step include identification of the apparent effect threshold (where one may exist) and/or the no-observed-adverse-effect level (NOAEL), identification of the slope of the dose-response curve (with appropriate confidence limits), and identification of the point or region of effect/response saturation.

Selection of the highest dose when the study objective is dose-response evaluation may not differ significantly from selection of the highest dose for hazard identification, although the goal of dose-response evaluation does not necessarily require the sensitivity of the assay to be maximized. When the shape or slope of the dose-response curve in the range of higher doses differs from the shape or slope of the curve in the range of lower doses, a high dose will not provide information on the curve at lower doses. In this case, of greater importance will be selection of lower doses that provide information on the shape or slope of the dose-response curve as well as the presence (if any) of an apparent threshold dose. However, the number of animals required to describe the dose-response curve at environmentally relevant doses may be prohibitively high and the shape of the dose-response curve may not be definable at these lower doses.

Exposure

Issues such as the level of human exposure expected from standard uses of a substance and the expected routes and scenarios of exposure may need to be considered during the dose- selection process for studies with the objective of safety determination. For example, administration by gavage may result in very high targe organ exposures, resulting in toxicity and other effects not observed when the compound is administered by inhalation or in the diet. Selection of doses to determine safety typically occurs for pharmaceuticals where potential exposure can readily be predicted based on prescribed intake (with appropriate variance). However, prediction of human exposure for widely used environmental chemicals (pesticides, industrial chemicals, etc.), may be much more difficult.

Selection of the highest dose, where the study objective is safety determination, may differ significantly from selection of the highest dose for hazard identification. For safety determination, the objective is to protect humans from potential toxic effects of a substance at typical exposure levels. The first step in this exercise is determination of the average and highest exposure levels. All potential exposure scenarios and routes (occupational, residential, environmental/ingestion, inhalation, dermal, etc.) should be considered to define average and highest potential exposures. Variability in human exposure as a function of age, gender, lifestyle, etc. also must be identified.

Once human exposure has been characterized, the highest dose may be selected as a multiple (e.g. 1×, 10×, 100×, 1000×, etc.) of that exposure, although concurrent consideration of the MTD also must occur. This approach may not account for very high human exposures that occur via accidents. Further, toxicity testing may need to be repeated if uses of the chemical change with a resultant increase in potential human exposure.

Dose Selection Based on Practical (Biological/Chemical) Considerations

A number of practical considerations, such as nutritional effects, physicochemical factors, and the bioavailability of the compound, will influence the selection of the highest dose for chronic rodent bioassays. It is common practice to select doses for chronic rodent bioassays that will minimize or avoid adverse nutritional effects. Such effects include disruption of the normal balance and availability of essential minerals, vitamins, fatty acids, etc. Adverse effects also may result from changes in the palatability of the medium (food or drinking water) either through physical modification or through organoleptic effects.

Physicochemical factors such as the solubility of the chemical in the vehicle (e.g., drinking water, corn oil, etc.), the vapor pressure of the substance (potential for volatilization), and the potential for interactions between the chemical and vehicle also may affect dose selection. Other considerations include the potential for the substance to cause concentration- or dose-specific adverse effects at the site of administration, such as erosion or ulceration (for dermal exposures) or irritation. There are also practical limits with regard to inhalation studies of particulates; that is, there is a limit to the amount of material that can be suspended.

The National Toxicology Program (NTP), as part of their assessment of factors limiting dose selection in 2-year animal bioassays (discussed in Chapter 2), assessed a variety of technical factors that tend to limit the amount of chemical that can be administered to an animal. These technical factors are typically important for relatively nontoxic substances and include consideration of issues such as the amount of chemical that can be delivered as a stable solution or suspension in a gavage vehicle. For dosed-feed studies, the percentage of the total weight of diet given to the animal was the primary factor limiting dose levels for 20% of the sex/species groups studied by this route of administration.

Poor palatability of dosed drinking water solutions or dosed feed can lead to the death of study animals. In instances when death or debilitation occurs from food or water rejection, animals frequently present with a characteristic pattern of lesions including cellular depletion in the thymus, spleen, lymph node, and bone marrow as well as testicular and ovarian atrophy. This problem rarely confounds dose selection because it is typically not encountered unless body-weight gains are markedly lower than controls or unless animals become moribund or lose weight during a study.

SELECTION OF THE MIDDLE AND LOWEST DOSES

Selection of middle doses facilitates an evaluation of the shape and slope of the dose-response curve. Particularly important is the selection of middle doses at levels that may induce disease by mechanisms different than those operative at the highest dose (this issue is discussed in more detail in the next chapter).

Early design specifications for the rodent cancer bioassay called for two dose groups plus controls (NTP 1984). Often the doses selected were the MTD and one-half the MTD. A rather close spacing of doses in two-dose studies afforded protection in the event that the top dose proved too high, resulting in poor survival. The second dose would be sufficiently close to the MTD to preserve the power of the assay to identify a carcinogen. With the increasing use of rodent cancer assay data in quantitative risk assessment, increasing importance was given to determining the shape of the dose-response curve. As a consequence, a third dose was added to the standard assay design. Eighty-two percent (242 of 296) of the experimental groups (individual sex/species combinations) in NTP studies designed from 1984 to 1994 were evaluated with three dose levels.

The third dose has proven to be valuable. Of the NTP studies of 49 chemicals that have undergone peer review between 1984 and 1994, there were 44 experimental groups (sex/species combinations) that were evaluated in three dose studies and showed a positive carcinogenic response. Of the 44 groups, 19 showed a statistically significant elevated tumor incidence at the low dose for at least one tumor that was considered chemically related. In 35 of the 44 experimental groups, there was an increase in the number of tumors in the third dose that, although not always statistically significant, nonetheless provided additional information about the shape of the dose-response curve.

Although the third dose is helpful in defining the shape of the dose-response curve, it must be pointed out that the overall range of doses in three-dose carcinogenicity studies is still limited. Figure 1 illustrates the spacing of doses used for the middle- and low-dose groups expressed as a function of the MTD; also shown is the number of experimental groups for which the various fractional doses were chosen.

The middle dose most often chosen was one-half or one-third of the MTD. Cases in which a lower fraction of the MTD was selected included some drugs that exerted a clear pharmacologic action at the top dose and instances when there was uncertainty over the potential for this action to affect survival with prolonged administration. In other instances, a somewhat lower middle dose was chosen based on the presence of a lesion of uncertain biological significance in a prechronic study and when the top dose of the cancer study was anticipated to cause this lesion.

Third doses were most often 1/4th or 1/10th of the MTD. For only 7 of 79 chemicals included in this data set was a third dose selected that was less than 1/10th of the MTD. These studies were some of the same in which the spacing was large between the top and middle dose. In some cases, a low dose was chosen to equal an effective blood concentration of a pharmaceutical or to equal an occupational exposure guideline.

The Interagency Staff Group on Carcinogens (ISGC 1986) suggests that the selection of middle doses should be based on the slope of the dose-response curve—a steep dose-response curve requires closer spacing of intermediate doses than a shallow dose-response curve. ISGC (1986) also suggests that the existence of metabolic saturation at doses below those identified by pathologic criteria suggest spacing of doses to determine carcinogenic potential (at the highest dose) as well as to define the dose-response curve for the saturable process. In some cases, such a determination may require more than two or three doses typically chosen for the chronic bioassay. Finally, the Committee on Carcinogenicity of Chemicals in Food, Consumer Products, and the Environment in the United Kingdom (1991) has suggested that the middle dose be set as the geometric mean of the highest and lowest doses.

Gaylor et al. (1985) suggest that, for linear dose-response relationships, the selection of middle doses makes little difference as long as a highest dose and controls are used. For sublinear dose-response relationships, doses below one-fourth to one-ninth of the highest dose generally result in tumor rates that are indistinguishable from the background rates in controls. Lower doses that produce tumor incidence rates within the background noise levels are relatively uninformative. To increase the power of middle doses to detect an ef-

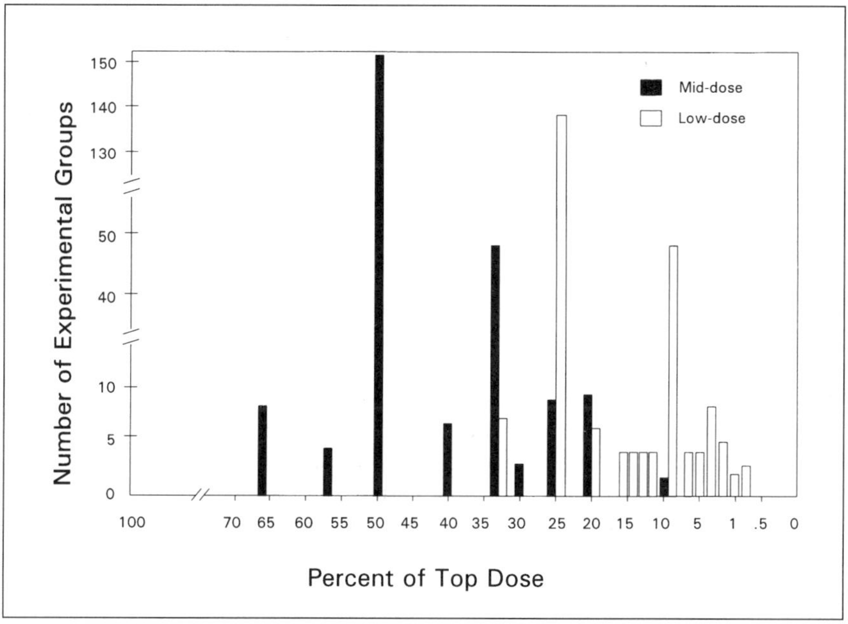

Figure 1. Dose spacing in NTP Carcinogenicity studies-1984–1994.

fect, it may be desirable to place more animals at doses that begin to show increases in disease above the background control rate; however, these doses may not be known before the chronic bioassay.

Some examples of the rationale for middle-dose selection can be drawn from the analysis of NTP bioassays. In selection of the concentrations for isobutene in a 2-year inhalation study, there were no lesions or changes in body-weight gains in prechronic studies that were considered of sufficient biologic importance on which to base dose selection. Therefore, the highest dose was selected based on flammable vapor concentration, whereas the middle-exposure concentration was set at the inflection point of a published biphasic curve of the kinetics of elimination of isobutene generated in gas-uptake studies. The lowest-exposure level was based on the lower linear (nonsaturated) portion of the kinetic curve.

As described in Chapter 2, NTP has begun to consider toxicokinetic data in conjunction with other prechronic study findings for dose selection. For example, when considering a chemical showing nonlinear or biphasic elimination kinetics, if other factors permit, the top dose for 2-year studies may be set above the inflection point in the "saturated" range. The middle doses then would be in the inflection area of the curve, and the lowest dose would be well down on the linear portion of the "nonsaturated" region.

A similar approach has been used for substances that induce cell proliferation (through, for example, cytotoxicity), where high and middle doses have been selected that do and do not cause proliferation and cytotoxicity, respectively. As discussed in Chapter 5, cell proliferation is a strong enhancer of the carcinogenic process. Genotoxic carcinogens will yield weaker responses below doses that produce regenerative cell proliferation, whereas nongenotoxic-cytotoxic carcinogens may have a threshold dose below which neither regenerative cell proliferation nor tumor incidence is increased. For a chemical that augments an ongoing biological process that influences tumorigenesis, e.g., mitogenesis, there may, however, not be a threshold dose (Olin et al. 1995). The presence of tumors in nonexposed control animals may indicate that endogenous and/or exogenous factors were sufficient to have already surpassed threshold doses. Hence, the addition of a chemical that augments an existing carcinogenic process will have an effect (Crump et al. 1976). A threshold dose under controlled experimental conditions may not be realized in a heterogeneous population exposed to a wide variety of environmental conditions.

Selection of the lowest dose may be based on the desire to identify a NOAEL for toxicity and/or cancer (where a carcinogenic threshold exists). Selection of the lowest dose also may be based on a multiple of human exposure (which may be either above or below an effect threshold) or a multiple of the NOAEL (where one has been identified). When justified scientifically, the lowest dose may be a fraction of the highest dose (as described by the NTP) or set at a level high enough to elicit an effect. Finally, the lowest dose may be influenced by the use of the benchmark dose approach (Barnes et al. 1995), which does not require the determination of a NOAEL.

SUMMARY

In this chapter, the factors that influence dose selection for chronic rodent bioassays have been examined. These factors include the objective of the bioassay as well as an array of practical (biological/chemical) considerations. Both study objective (hazard identification, dose-response evaluation, exposure evaluation) and practical considerations may be particularly influential on selection of the highest dose. Issues such as study sensitivity, elicitation of toxicity, mechanistic concurrence between high and lower doses, and human exposure as well as issues such as nutritional effects, physicochemical factors, and the bioavailability of the compound are critical considerations in selection of the highest dose. Selection of the middle and lower doses will be influenced by the desire to examine the shape of the dose-response curve, to identify effects at or near potential human exposures, or to identify NOAELs.

There has been considerable discussion of the selection of the highest dose in assays for carcinogenicity that elicit cancer by mechanisms that may not be operable at lower doses or exposure levels (NTP 1992, McConnell 1995, Swenberg 1995, Counts and Goodman 1995). Detailed examinations of this issue are presented in the next chapter through a series of chemical-specific case studies.

REFERENCES

Barnes DG, Daston GP, Evans JS, et al. (1995) Criteria for use of a benchmark dose to estimate a reference dose. Reg Toxicol Pharmacol 21:296–306

Committee on Carcinogenicity of Chemicals in Food, Consumer Products and the Environment (COC) (1991) Guidelines for the Evaluation of Chemicals for Carcinogenicity. Report No. 42 on Health and Social Subjects. Department of Health, London

Counts JL, Goodman JI (1995) Principles underlying dose selection for, and extrapolation from, the carcinogen bioassay: Dose influences mechanism. Reg Toxicol Pharmacol 21:418–421

Crump KS, Hoel DG, Langley CH, Peto R (1976) Fundamental carcinogenic processes and their implications for low dose risk assessment. Cancer Res 2973–2979

Davies D (1992) Dose levels—how should they be selected and what is the role of pharmacokinetics? An Academic/regulatory viewpoint. In McAuslane JAN, Lumley CE, Walker SR (eds), The Carcinogenicity Debate, CMR Workshop Series. Quay, Lancaster, UK, pp 159–164

Gaylor DW, Chen JJ, Kodell RL (1985) Experimental design of bioassays for screening and low dose extrapolation. Risk Analysis 5:9–16

Haseman JK (1985) Issues in carcinogenicity testing: Dose selection. Fundam Appl Toxicol 5:67–78

Huff J, Rall DP (1992) Relevance to humans of carcinogenesis results from laboratory animals toxicology studies. In Last JM, Wallace RB (eds), Maxcy-Rosenau-Last Public Health and Preventative Medicine, 13th ed. Appleton & Lange, Norwalk, CT, pp 433–440 and 453–457

Interagency Staff Group on Carcinogens (ISGC) (1986) Chemical carcinogens: A review of the science and its associated principles. Environ Health Perspec 67:201–282

International Conference on Harmonisation (ICH) of Technical Requirements for Registration of Pharmaceuticals for Human Use (1995) Fed Register 60:11278, March

McConnell EE (1995) Historical review of the rodent bioassay and future directions. Reg Toxicol Pharmacol 21:38–43

National Research Council (1983) Risk Assessment in the Federal Government: Managing the Process. National Academy Press, Washington, DC

National Research Council (1993) Use of the maximum tolerated dose in animal bioassays for carcinogenicity. In Goldstein B et al. (eds), Issues in Risk Assessment. National Academy Press, Washington, DC, pp 15–83

National Toxicology Program—Board of Scientific Counselors (1984) Report of the NTP ad hoc panel on chemical carcinogenesis testing and evaluation. Department of Health and Human Services, Washington, DC

National Toxicology Program—Board of Scientific Counselors (1992) Final Report of the Advisory Review. Fed Register 57:31721–31730. July 17

Olin S, Farland W, Park C, Rhomberg L, Scheuplein R, Starr T, Wilson J, eds (1995) Low-dose extrapolation of cancer risks: issues and perspectives. ILSI Press, Washington, DC

Swenberg JA (1995) Bioassay design and MTD setting: Old methods and new approaches. Reg Toxicol Pharmacol 21:44–51

Usui T (1992) Dose levels—how should they be selected and what is the role of pharmacokinetics? An industry viewpoint. In McAuslane JAN, Lumley CE, Walker SR (eds), The Carcinogenicity Debate. CMR Workshop Series. Quay, Lancaster, UK, pp 165–178

Weissinger J (1992) Dose levels—how should they be selected and what is the role of pharmacokinetics? A regulatory viewpoint. In McAuslane JAN, Lumley CE, Walker SR (eds), The Carcinogenicity Debate. CMR Workshop Series. Quay, Lancaster, UK, pp 147–153

Chapter 5

Mechanistic Issues in Dose Selection

SELECTING DOSES FOR GENOTOXIC COMPOUNDS[1]

Introduction

The fact that electrophiles are reactive to nucleophiles such as DNA and proteins means that a variety of chemical/biological information can be applied to the prediction of macromolecular chemical adduction. For the DNA-reactive (genotoxic) chemical carcinogens there exists a strong association between potential or actual electrophilic centers in the molecule, DNA-reactivity, mutagenicity in vitro and in vivo, and transpecies/multiple site carcinogenicity. This confluence of properties is shown at the top of Figure 1. As also shown in Figure 1, with the passage of time an increasing number of rodent carcinogens have been defined that break, in one way or another, this paradigm of genotoxic carcinogenesis. Despite the many inadequacies of the term, these latter carcinogens have become known as nongenotoxic carcinogens. At the bottom of Figure 1 it is implied that the formal separation of these two classes of carcinogens is useful at the extremes, e.g., sodium saccharin compared to benzo[*a*]pyrene, but the polarization is complicated by the fact that both genotoxic and nongenotoxic influences are intrinsic to the induction of tumors in rodents. Nonetheless, the poles in Figure 1 are recognizable, together with an area of overlap—these three areas are shown by example in Figure 2. In Figure 2, limonene is used to illustrate the purest form of nongenotoxic carcinogenesis, glycidol is used to illustrate overt genotoxic carcinogenesis, and the Wyeth peroxisome proliferator is used to illustrate a rodent liver carcinogen that probably induces tumors by a nongenotoxic mechanism, but genotoxic influences such as clastogenesis cannot be excluded.

Distinction of Genotoxic and Nongenotoxic Carcinogenicity

The brief introduction above illustrates the fact that there is no simple divide between genotoxic and nongenotoxic carcinogenesis. The best that can be achieved is to gather appropriate data that will be useful for predicting likely rodent carcinogenicity for a chemical or for elucidating its major mechanism

---

[1] Contributed by John Ashby.

of carcinogenic action. Using the polar examples of limonene (Anon 1990a) and glycidol (Anon 1990b; Figure 2) enables the potential value of consideration of genotoxicity to be illustrated. Thus, glycidol is naturally electrophilic and displays genetic toxicity with the first assay conducted—the *Salmonella* test (Anon 1990b). The more tests that are conducted on glycidol, the more

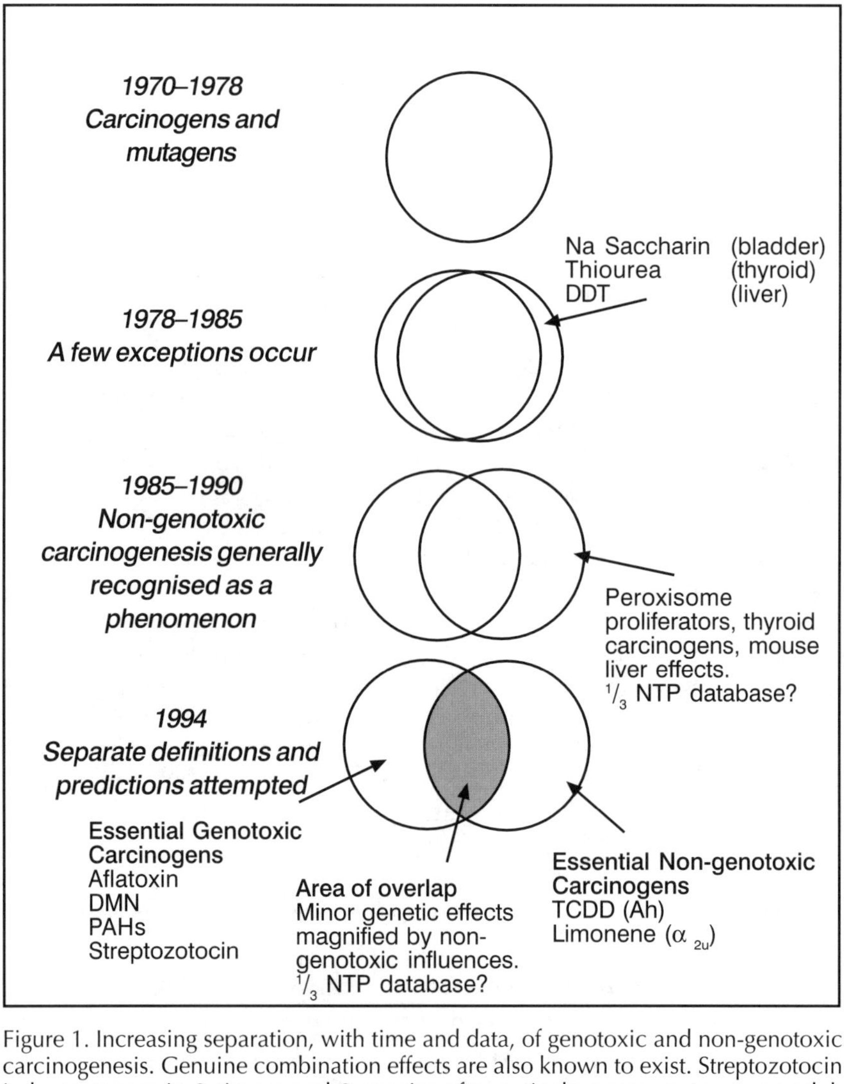

Figure 1. Increasing separation, with time and data, of genotoxic and non-genotoxic carcinogenesis. Genuine combination effects are also known to exist. Streptozotocin induces cancer in 3 tissues and 3 species after a single exposure to young adult animals illustrating essential genotoxic carcinogenesis. NTP = US National Toxicology Program rodent carcinogenicity database.

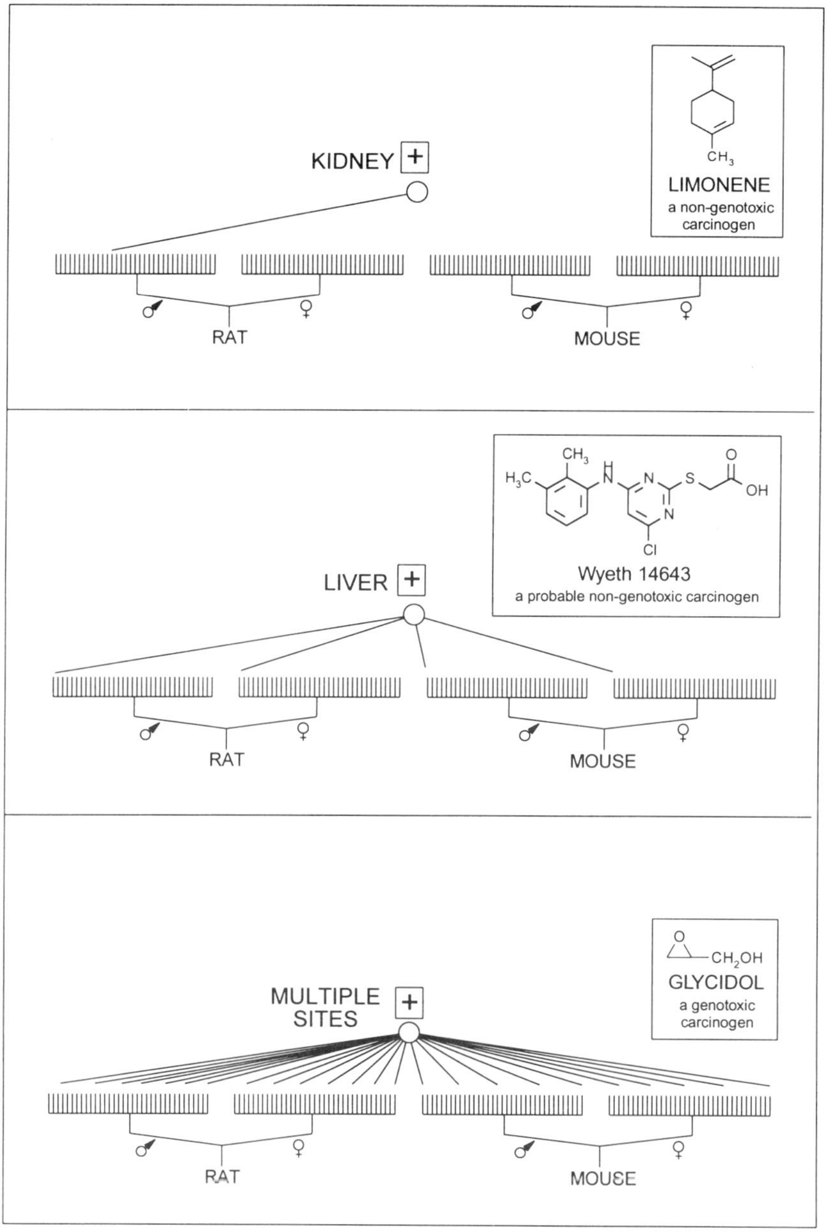

Figure 2. In routine rodent carcinogenicity bioassays it is usual to assess at least 35 tissues from each animal. Limonene affects only the male rat kidney, Wyeth 14643 the rodent liver, and glycidol a total of 24 sites among mice and rats. Each chemical can be referred to as a 'rodent carcinogen'.

evidence that accrues to indicate its intrinsic eletrophilicity and genetic toxicity (Anon 1990b). Having established intrinsic electrophilicity for glycidol, secondary questions such as its most favored sites of reactivity on DNA can be considered. Thus, chemicals that preferentially alkylate the O^6 group of guanosine are more likely to induce cancer than are agents that attack the N-7 group of guanosine. Vogel (1989) has discussed these secondary criteria in detail, and at their best they enable an initial alert to carcinogenicity to be accentuated or attenuated (e.g., for methylnitrosourea and methyl chloride, respectively). Observation of genetic toxicity for a chemical, particularly in vivo, is a strong indication of its potential genotoxic carcinogenicity.

Limonene provides contrary indications. The chemical itself is nonmutagenic in the primary genetic toxicity assays, and this includes assessments of the epoxide derivatives that may be formed metabolically from its two isolated ethylenic double bonds (Anon 1990a). Evaluation of limonene in rodents reveals the one outstanding property of renal necrosis and compensatory renal cell division—effects initiated by precipitation of specific protein complexes in the kidneys of male rats (Goldsworthy et al. 1987, Swenberg 1993). Limonene therefore presents clear potential to be a tissue- and rodent-specific nongenotoxic carcinogen, but it has little or no potential for genotoxic carcinogenesis.

The above contrast between glycidol and limonene suggests that one must seek reasons why glycidol should not be carcinogenic to humans and why limonene should be. This subtle distinction can have a profound influence on carcinogen risk analysis.

The Role of Induced Cell Division in Chemical Carcinogenicity

Supplement 5 of Volume 101 of *Environmental Health Perspectives* deals in detail with the role of induced cell division in chemical carcinogenicity. Although there is general agreement that a one-to-one relationship between these two phenomena does not exist, there are also many lines of evidence favoring the idea that induction of cell division by a nongenotoxic carcinogen is probably a critical etiologic event in certain tissues of rodents. Several authors in Supplement 5 note, critical to this discussion, that the chemical adduction of DNA by a genotoxin may have no threshold dose level, whereas stimulation of cell division in response to induced biological changes will have a threshold dose. The central point therefore emerges that, if a chemical is overtly genotoxic, the prospects for a no-effect dose level (threshold) are reduced to consideration of the statistical resolving power of the cancer bioassay. If, however, genotoxicity can be essentially eliminated, any carcinogenic activities shown by the chemical are likely to be dominated by threshold-related biological disturbances induced in rodents and accompanied by secondary cell division. In such cases, selection of dose levels in cancer bioassays based on the level of biological disturbance should enable the demonstration of an absolute threshold dose level (Ashby and Morrod 1991). Examples of dose selection for nongenotoxic (threshold acting) toxicants are provided later in this chapter.

The absence of a general and clear distinction between genotoxicity and nongenotoxicity for all chemicals (see Figures 1 and 2) implies that individual chemicals must be considered in isolation and judgment exercised as to their intrinsic genetic toxicity (Butterworth 1990, Perera 1991, Ashby and Tennant 1994). The major steps in this process are as follows.

Measurement of Genetic Toxicity

Chemical Structure

The key structural features associated with direct or metabolism-dependent electrophilicity in chemicals have been listed (Miller and Miller 1977, Ashby 1994a). Such structural features provide a major, but nondefinitive, indicator of potential genotoxicity for a chemical.

Genetic Toxicity Observed in Vitro

Despite residual discussions, there is now general agreement that the intrinsic genetic toxicity of a chemical can be assessed by the adequate conduct of two or three in vitro genetic toxicity assays. The usual practice is to assess a chemical by the *Salmonella* assay, an assay for the induction of chromosomal aberrations, and an assay for genetic toxicity at a named gene—most usually the *tk* locus of mouse lymphoma L5178Y cells. Assessment of such data usually leads to a clear indication of agents' genetic toxicity, but value judgments may be required to derive a clear conclusion. These judgments include consideration of the significance of isolated positive responses, weak positive responses, and positive responses observed only at toxic dose levels. Some scientists believe that the conduct of further supplementary in vitro assays is of little value in reaching a conclusion of genetic toxicity not apparent after the conduct of the primary assays. Staying with the chemicals shown in Figure 2, glycidol would be rapidly established as genotoxic, limonene as nongenotoxic, and the Wyeth compound as possessed of selective genetic toxicities (Lefevre et al. 1994). Experience has shown that the conduct of further genetic toxicity tests would not refine these conclusions (Tennant et al. 1987).

Genetic Toxicity Observed in Vivo

When a chemical elicits clear evidence of genetic toxicity in rodents, this has a major influence on predicting or explaining its carcinogenicity. In particular, genetic toxicity observed in vivo substantially weakens the prospect of nongenotoxic carcinogenesis. Such data do not exclude nongenotoxic carcinogenesis, but they mandate that significant mechanistic studies must be derived to overrule the assumption of genotoxic carcinogenesis. The potent genetic toxicity of the large majority of human carcinogens and the reference (genotoxic) rodent carcinogens in primary rodent genetic toxicity assays support this assumption (Ashby and Tinwell 1994). The mouse bone marrow micronucleus assay is the primary rodent genetic toxicity assay, but additional use is made of assays such as the rat liver DNA repair assay, the mouse coat color spot test, ^{32}P-postlabeling, and, recently, transgenic mouse mutation assays.

A major current concern derives from our present level of uncertainty regarding the extent of nongenotoxic carcinogens in the literature. For example, the apparent low sensitivity of the mouse bone marrow micronucleus assay to twenty-four of the National Toxicology Program (NTP) rodent carcinogens (Shelby et al. 1993) poses the underlying question of how many of these carcinogens are operating primarily via a nongenotoxic mechanism (Ashby and Tinwell 1994). At the moment, there are no clear answers to such questions—judgment must again prevail. What is now certain is that the simple paradigm that carcinogenesis and mutagenesis are interchangeable terms is no longer valid.

Selection of Dose Levels for in Vivo Genetic Toxicity Assay

Before considering dose-level selection for rodent cancer bioassays, it is pertinent to note that much confusion also exists in dose selection for short-term rodent genetic toxicity experiments. As with cancer bioassays, a mistaken idea persists that high-dose levels can compensate for the use of small groups of test animals. That argument implies a simple linear relationship between dose and effect—a condition rarely encountered. Thus, at high-dose levels one often encounters *new* toxicities, not necessarily *amplified* toxicity. The classic example of acetaminophen toxicity to the liver is shown in Figure 3. It is only when glutathione levels are reduced by gavage dosing of acetaminophen that protein binding commences. Similar daily dose levels spread over 12 hours (in diet) are noncarcinogenic, despite the alert provided by the acute gavage data. It is clear that the high-dose acute data on protein binding provide no relevant information regarding the carcinogenic hazard of acetaminophen administered in the diet. This dislocation between the two observations is indicated by the threshold nature of the acute protein binding (Figure 3).

Another complication of acute rodent genetic toxicity experiments is that the test animals usually are sampled within 24 hours of dosing. This means that dose levels that would be lethal over a few days can be used in experi-

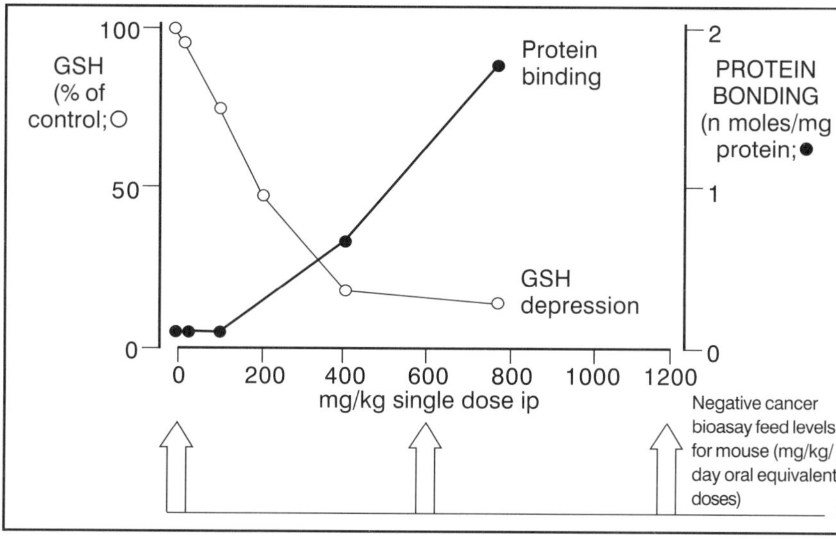

Figure 3. Acute oral gavage dosing toxicity of acetaminophen to the mouse liver, and gavage dose equivalents of the negative dietary mouse cancer bioassay. (Mitchell et al. 1973 and Anon. 1993b, respectively).

ments terminated within 24 hours. This practice can make the difference between a positive and a negative assay result, as shown for dimethylnitrosamine (DMN) in Figure 4. The advent of transgenic rodent mutation assays has forced consideration of the delayed death phenomenon simply because such animals must survive 7 to 14 days after dosing to allow for mutation fixation.

In vivo genetic toxicity data are suggested here to play an important role in carcinogenicity prediction, so it is relevant to note that the issues surrounding cancer bioassay dose-level selection have a strong echo in acute genetic toxicity assay dose selection.

Selection of Dose Levels for Rodent Carcinogenicity Bioassays

This much-discussed subject usually devolves to a discussion of whether or not to use the maximum tolerated dose (MTD) as the highest-dose level. Proponents of use of the MTD usually emphasize the need for enhanced assay sensitivity. Detractors of the use of the MTD usually question the relevance to humans of the high-dose test data. The reasons why the debate continues are 2-fold. First, statistical resolving power of the bioassay is, in fact, a real problem because large group sizes become prohibitively expensive. Second, setting the top dose level without reference to the MTD can become dangerously arbitrary. In fact, there is no simple answer to the high-dose issue, as will be

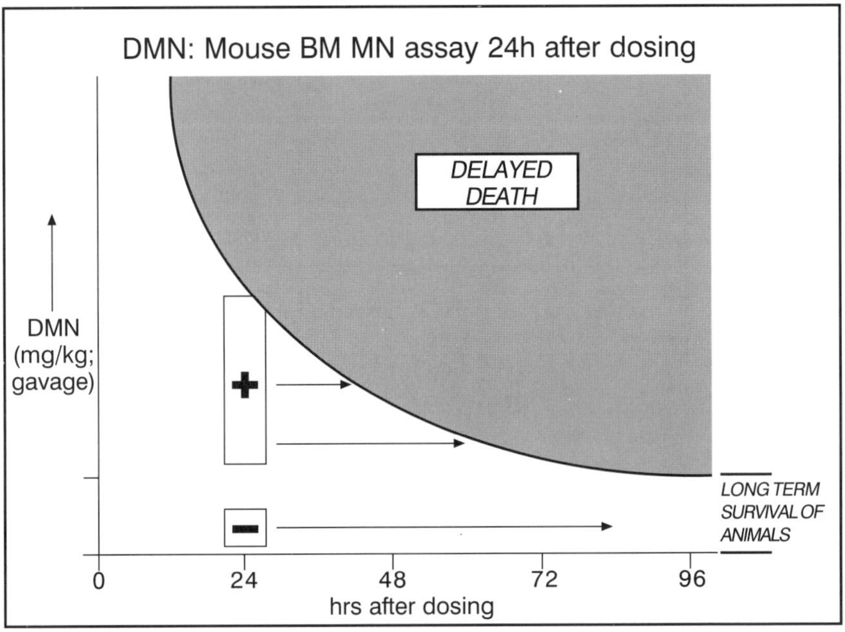

Figure 4. Demonstration of inactivity in a 24 hour mouse bone marrow micronucleus assay (BM MN) for dose-levels of dimethylnitrosamine (DMN) that would be compatible with the long term survival of the test animals. At higher dose-levels a positive response in the MN assay can be observed at the 24h sampling time, but such animals would eventually have died (based on Morrison and Ashby 1994).

illustrated here. One has to become acquainted with the characteristics of the test chemical and then pose a precise question regarding its carcinogenic potential, itself framed within the context of the ways in which humans may come into contact with the material.

Haseman and Lockhart (1994) have reviewed the NTP rodent carcinogenicity database and shown that a negligible proportion of the carcinogens are carcinogenic only at the highest dose. The only problem with that statement is that the next-lower dose level is within a small factor of the highest dose; it may therefore be that the real issue under discussion is the highest dose and dose levels within a factor of 2 of it. The Haseman and Lockhart (1994) analysis also shows that the extent (across species) of carcinogenicity of a chemical is broadly related to its electrophilic potential (Figure 5). Somewhat consistent with this is the analysis of the rodent carcinogenicity of the human carcinogens, as reported by Apostolou (1990). There it was shown (Figure 6) that it is not necessary to use the MTD in rodents for bioassays of human carcinogens. That conclusion also is suspect because we are aware of only the relatively potent human carcinogens because of the statistical limitations

Rat		Mouse		Salmonella +ve(%)	No. in group
Male	Female	Male	Female		
At least one mouse gender and one rat gender with 2 dose groups statistically elevated over controls				76	45
All four test groups having one or both dose groups statistically elevated over controls				73.5	34
Only one of four test groups with two dose groups statistically elevated over controls				42.5	41
Two of the four test groups giving no evidence (NE) of carcinogenicity				47	74
Two of the four test groups giving no evidence or equivocal evidence of carcinogenicity				45	95

Figure 5. Re-presentation of the data of Haseman and Lockhart (1994). The level of carcinogenic activity in rodents (across the four test groups considering dose-response) for the NTP agents studied by Haseman and Lockhart has been broken into the five groups shown. For each of these groups, the number of test agents in the group, and the percentage that are mutagenic to Salmonella, are shown. Activity in the Salmonella assay correlates with the ability of the carcinogen to produce tumours at sub-MTD dose-levels and in more than two of the four test groups. Also, to have at least two of the four test groups with no or equivocal evidence of carcinogenicity correlates with inactivity in the Salmonella assay.

of human epidemiologic studies. Nonetheless, these two studies (Haseman and Lockhart 1994, Apostolou 1990) suggest that a simple rejection of the MTD is not possible.

Each of the stages in the carcinogenesis process is subject to different controlling influences. It is these influences that deserve careful attention when deciding on the dose levels to use in a rodent cancer bioassay. The simplest two-stage model available, covalent addition of the test agent to DNA followed by cell division to transform the adducted base into a mutant base, illustrates how one event (adduction) may well be linear with dose, whereas stimulation of cell division may be mechanistically independent of the first step and nonlinear with respect to dose.

Mirsalis et al. (1994) have discussed this simple two-stage model within the context of the expression of mutations in the livers of transgenic mice exposed to DMN. Likewise, Goldsworthy et al. (1987) have discussed the renal carcinogenicity of limonene within a similar context. It follows from

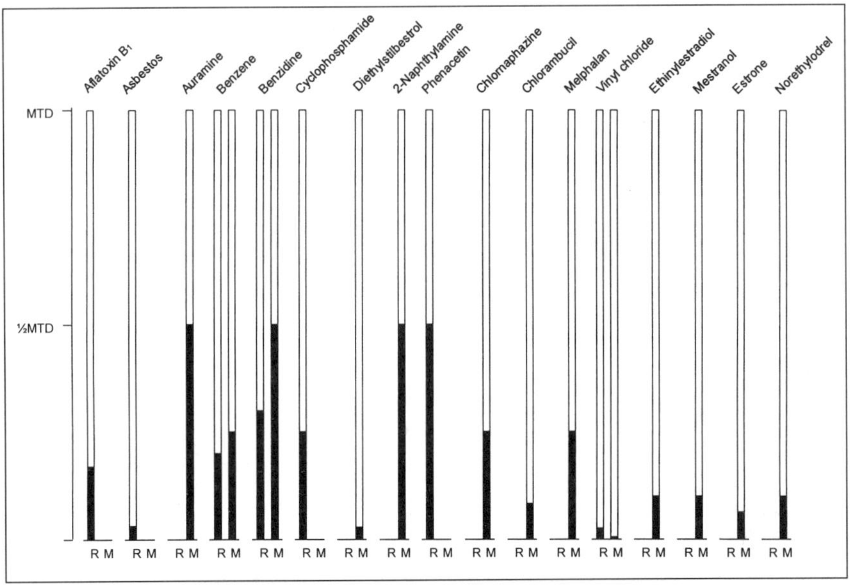

Figure 6. Representation of data of Apostolou (1990) regarding established human carcinogens where carcinogenicity to rodents is known and where the rodent bioassay dose-levels have been correlated with the maximum tolerated dose (MTD) of the chemical. R = rat, M = mouse. The height of the black bar represents the lowest dose (fraction of MTD) at which a statistically significant elevation of tumour bearing animals occurs.

these simple examples that the individual dosimetry of any one of the many mechanistically distinct stages of carcinogenesis can become the primary determinant of the eventual production of tumors in a bioassay. The manner in which the test agent is administered also can affect peak blood levels of the chemical, which in turn may modify in a critical way one or more of the stages of carcinogenesis. The level of complexity is unlikely ever to submit to a simple and single rule for dose selection, as is illustrated by the two NTP rodent bioassays of benzyl acetate.

The history of the bioassays of benzyl acetate is shown in Figure 7. It is essentially nongenotoxic and the original gavage bioassay yielded evidence of carcinogenicity at three sites. However, uncertainty accompanied each of these instances of cancer induction. Use of a nonirritant dose level probably would have eliminated the tumors of the forestomach. The corn oil vehicle probably was responsible for the pancreatic tumors, and adenomas in the mouse liver are unexceptional. A repeat bioassay conducted in feed was negative. In the second NTP Technical Report (Anon 1993a) it was noted that peak blood levels of benzoic acid, a primary hydrolysis/metabolic product of benzyl acetate was 300 times higher in the gavage study than in the feed study. Thus,

NTP Tech. Report No. (year)	Genetic Toxicity	Route of administration	Top dose-level		Neoplastic Findings	Comments
			Rat	Mouse		
250 (1986)	3 assays -ve L5178Y +ve	gavage	500 mg/kg	1000 mg/kg	Male rat. Pancreatic adenomas Mice. Liver adenomas, forestomach adenomas/carcinomas	Corn oil vehicle contributed to pancreatic effects? Local irritation contributed to stomach effects? Peak blood levels of benzoic acid ~300x higher than in feed study
431 (1993)	Additionally; 4 mouse assays -ve drosophila -ve	feed	12,000ppm (~550 mg/kg/d)	3000ppm (~350 mg/kg/d)	Non-carcinogenic	Palatability established top dose level in rat.

Figure 7. Major characteristics and findings of the NTP carcinogenicity bioassays of benzyl acetate, as abstracted by Ashby (1994b). +ve = positive in assay, -ve = negative in assay.

the central issue was not the use of the MTD but rather use of a dosing regimen that could amplify the highest dose by approximately 300 times. Curiously, the rat feed study did not achieve a MTD because of lack of palatability—itself not considered by the NTP to be a meaningful measure of a high dose. Benzyl acetate therefore illustrates the toxicologic concepts that are most relevant to dose/route selection. First, the agent is nonelectrophilic and nongenotoxic in vitro and in vivo. This powerful information was accrued only during the course of the bioassays. Second, if a bioassay were to be conducted, attention should have been focused on the route of exposure. As a food additive/perfumery agent, use of feed or skin painting studies would be indicated. Under such test conditions, a carcinogenic hazard would not be indicated.

Selection of bioassay dose levels for both genotoxic and nongenotoxic compounds should therefore derive from an holistic appraisal of the chemistry and toxicology of the test chemical. The dosimetry of obvious toxicities will probably influence the bioassay outcome, and this forces the question back to why the bioassay is being conducted. Faccini et al. (1992) have captured the complex process of dose selection as follows:

> This will be based on pre-existing toxicity studies including toxicokinetics and in the absence of previous toxicity testing, usually on a specific 3-month study. This study should allow the calculation of the putative high, medium, and low doses on the basis of clinical and pathological parameters.
>
> On the one hand, the high dose should be the maximum which does not induce a direct toxic effect, for example, liver parenchymatous single cell necrosis and on the other hand, pharmacological effects and adaptive changes such as increased volume of the liver or adrenals are acceptable as well as behavioral changes such as decreased activity.
>
> The low dose should be some multiple of the anticipated human exposure providing that the bioavailability of the test agent appears to be in the same range for both animal species and man.
>
> The intermediate dose could be in geometric progression between the other two doses allowing for the calculation of a dose-effect relationship.

Summary

Assessment of the genetic toxicity of a chemical can be achieved by the use of well-established genetic toxicity assays. Observations made in rodents are of greater predictive/ mechanistic significance than effects constrained to cells cultured in vitro. All chemicals show some level of genetic toxicity if a sufficient number of assays are conducted, especially if toxic dose levels are

Parameter	Fotemustine	Vitamin C
Chemical structure	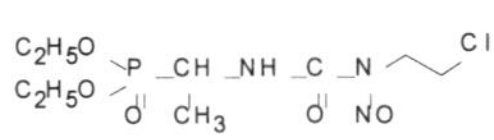	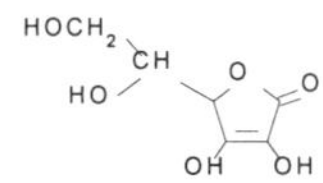
Chemical reactivity	electrophilic	non-electrophilic
Metabolism	possible formation of additional electrophiles	anti-oxidant, radical scavenger
Salmonella assay	+	-
Mouse BM MN assay		
a) Qualitative response	+	+
b) min. positive dose	16μmole/kg	2800μmole/kg
c) max. fold incr.	11x	3x
Source of MN assay activity	alkylation of DNA	radical damage to DNA following metabolic overload (?)
Carcinogenic potential to humans	+	-

Figure 8. Illustration of the synthesis of data required to discern the differential hazard to humans of two agents active in the mouse bone marrow micronucleus (BM MN) assay (from Tinwell and Ashby, 1994).

used. As a consequence, the greatest aid to an assessment of the genetic toxicity and carcinogenic potential of a chemical is judgment, as illustrated in Figure 8. Some chemicals are overtly genotoxic and this reflects heavily on their potential or actual carcinogenicity. In contrast, other chemicals are essentially devoid of genetic toxicity, and any carcinogenicity they display in rodents must be considered as arising via nongenetic tissue disturbances associated, at some stage, with induced cell division. In between are chemicals that induce tumors in rodents probably via subtle interactions of both genetic and nongenetic toxicities.

Ames and Gold (1990) have noted that half of all chemicals tested are carcinogenic to rodents, a finding reflected in pharmaceutical drugs (Davies and Monro 1995). Genetic toxicity is an important contributory influence to some of these carcinogens, but the driving force for many appears to be nongenetic toxicities of the chemicals. The dosimetry of these nongenetic toxicities (discussed later in this chapter) is the primary tool for selection of dose levels in rodent cancer bioassays.

Dose selection for genotoxic compounds requires consideration of information on structure, acute toxicity, the route of exposure, level of human exposure, and other issues. Of course, the frequency and duration of dosing will also modify any eventual tumorigenic responses. Some of these influences on carcinogenicity are caught in the envelope of the MTD, but the MTD itself is probably too blunt an index to use for setting dose levels. In fact, there is no simple prescriptive solution to the problem of bioassay dose setting for genotoxic compounds. The issues that must be considered are individual to each chemical and to the likely extent of human exposure to the chemical. The best general advice on dose setting for genotoxic compounds is, therefore, that of Faccini et al. (1992) repeated earlier.

THE USE OF INDUCED CELL PROLIFERATION IN SELECTING DOSES FOR CARCINOGENICITY STUDIES[2]

Cell Proliferation in Initiation

Cell Replication Enhances the Effectiveness of Mutagens

Cell division is required to convert a DNA adduct to a permanent mutation (Cayama et al. 1978). A genotoxic chemical administered at a toxic dose that also induces cell proliferation is far more effective as a mutagen and as a carcinogen than when given at a low dose that does not induce cell proliferation (Columbano et al. 1981). In a population of proliferating cells, there is less time for DNA repair processes to remove DNA adducts before cell replication converts adducts to mutations (Richardson et al. 1986).

In initiation/promotion protocols, animals are initiated by treatment with a mutagen *and* a regimen that induces cell proliferation (e.g., partial hepatectomy or neonatal liver growth) to enhance the effectiveness of the mutagen. For example, studies with the highly mutagenic, tobacco-specific nitrosamine 4-(*N*-methyl-*N*-nitrosamino)-1-(3-pyridyl)-1-butanone indicate that a quantitation of both promutagenic DNA adducts and cell proliferation secondary to toxicity are required to account for the site-specific nature of malignant tumor formation within the rat nose (Belinsky et al. 1987). Knowledge of cytotoxicity and cell proliferation as well as knowledge of the delivered dose to the target cells as assessed by DNA adduct formation provides a far more realistic risk assessment calculation than when only the administered dose of the chemical is considered (Belinsky et al. 1987, Hoel et al. 1983, Casanova et al. 1989, Starr 1989).

Mutations Occur As Events Secondary to Cell Proliferation

Enhanced cell replication also may increase the frequency of spontaneous and chemically associated mutations, either by errors in replication or by conversion of endogenous or exogenous DNA adducts to mutations before DNA repair can occur (Stott et al. 1981). Events of nondisjunction and mitotic recombination that can occur during cell division are effective in converting a heterozygous mutation to homozygosity or hemizygosity. Increased rates of cell replication associated with clonal expansion of lymphocyte populations in human subjects have been demonstrated to increase the mutant frequency in those clones (Allegretta et al. 1990). The possibility of mutational events oc-

---

[2] Contributed by Byron Butterworth, Michael Templin, Jeffery Larson, Douglas Wolf, and Thomas Goldsworthy (all of the Chemical Industry Institute of Toxicology).

curring in growth control genes is enhanced during replication because many of those genes are being transcribed as the cell cycles and may experience greater exposure to endogenous and exogenous mutagens (Fausto and Shank 1983, Bailey et al. 1989, Bailey et al. 1990, Braun et al. 1988, Mead and Fausto 1989). Similarly, mutations in DNA polymerases or DNA repair genes that are expressed in response to toxicity may lead to a cell exhibiting a mutator phenotype (Loeb 1991).

Cell Proliferation in Lesion Development

Mitogen-Induced Cell Proliferation in Promotion

Mitogenic agents are tissue specific and have been characterized best in the liver (reviewed by Loury et al. 1987). For the liver mitogens, there is a direct stimulation of cell division in the absence of chemically induced hepatic necrosis, as determined by microscopic examination and by the absence of liver-associated enzymes in the serum. Continued exposure to these agents induces hepatomegaly and a sustained increase in liver weight. Treatment with some mitogens can result in more than a doubling in liver weight. After the initial burst of cell proliferation associated with liver growth, the rate of cell turnover frequently returns to normal after the liver has reached its new size. With continued treatment, an increase in the number of hepatic preneoplastic foci is often seen as well as a substantial elevation in cell turnover within those foci. Examples of such agents are phenobarbital, α-hexachlorocyclohexane, polybrominated biphenyls, butylhydroxytoluene, ethinyl estradiol, cyproterone acetate, and most chemicals that also induce peroxisomal proliferation (Schulte-Hermann et al. 1983, Schroter et al. 1987, Schulte-Hermann et al. 1988, Cattley and Popp 1989).

Mitogenic agents have the ability to directly stimulate cell proliferation and often appear to act through a cellular receptor. Liver mitogens such as phenobarbital and α-hexachlorocyclohexane induce a hyperplastic increase in liver weight that is maintained with continued administration of the compound (Schulte-Hermann et al. 1983, Schroter et al. 1987, Schulte-Hermann et al. 1988). The carcinogenic activity of these compounds is dependent on continued administration of the agent, suggesting that altered growth control may be playing the critical role in tumor formation (Goldsworthy et al. 1986).

Homeostasis in normal tissue and growth of preneoplastic foci are characterized by the ratio of the rate of cell birth to the rate of cell death. Evidence to date indicates that mitogenic agents can cause the preferential growth of preneoplastic foci by altering the rates of cell birth and death (Cattley and Popp 1989, Marsman and Popp 1989).

Regenerative Cell Proliferation in Initiation and Promotion

Cytotoxicants induce necrosis and regenerative cell proliferation. Mutations may be induced secondary to the continual state of necrosis, inflammation, release of nucleases, and regenerative cell proliferation. In some cases, preferential growth of preneoplastic lesions may occur because cells in those lesions are more refractory to the cytotoxic effects of the agent relative to normal cells (Farber 1980). Additionally, preneoplastic cells may respond to the growth stimulatory signals associated with regeneration. Examples of carcinogens that appear to be acting through a nongenotoxic-cytotoxic mode of action are *d*-limonene in the male rat kidney, saccharin in the rat bladder, and carbon tetrachloride and chloroform in the rodent liver (Doolittle et al. 1987, Cohen and Ellwein 1990, Reitz et al. 1990, Flamm and Lehman-McKeeman 1991, Larson et al. 1994).

Events associated with regenerative cell proliferation induced by cytotoxicants may both increase the mutational frequency and also act as a stimulus for the preferential growth of precancerous or cancerous cells. Simple abrasion of the skin with a felt wheel to remove epidermal cells results in cell proliferation and is a strong promoting stimulus in the mouse skin two-stage carcinogenesis model (Argyris 1980, 1989). A greater susceptibility of normal cells to the cytotoxic effects of a compound relative to preneoplastic cells would also result in the preferential growth of those preneoplastic cells (Farber 1980). Several examples follow.

α_{2u}-Globulin-Mediated Male Rat Kidney Carcinogens

For many nongenotoxic renal carcinogens including unleaded gasoline, *d*-limonene, 1,4-dichlorobenzene, and pentachloroethane, tumor induction occurs in the kidneys of male but not female rats and in mice of either sex. The proposed mechanism of action for these agents is chemically induced accumulation of a male rat-specific protein, α_{2u}-globulin, in the form of protein droplets in the kidney tubule cells. This protein accumulation then results in cell death and regenerative cell proliferation (Borghoff et al. 1990, Flamm and Lehman-McKeeman 1991). The accumulation of α_{2u}-globulin-containing protein droplets and increased cell turnover have been shown to correlate with tumor formation in a dose-dependent and site-specific manner. Like the appearance of tumors, the protein accumulation and cell proliferation are seen in the kidneys of male rats only. Thus, regenerative cell proliferation and tumor formation are closely associated for this group of carcinogens (U.S. Environmental Protection Agency [EPA] 1991).

Terephthalic Acid

Another group of cytotoxic agents includes uracil and terephthalic acid. These chemicals yield urinary calculi and, in turn, produce a foreign body reaction with resulting hyperplasia of the bladder epithelium (Heck 1987). For these chemicals, relatively large doses of over 1% in the diet must be administered for long periods to exhibit promotional effects or production of papillomas or cancer. The primary action of these compounds appears to be production of bladder hyperplasia at the site where tumors eventually arise.

Chloroform

The strength of the evidence that chloroform is acting through a nongenotoxic-cytotoxic mode of action rests on the fact that chloroform lacks genotoxic activity and the observation of preceding cytotoxicity and regenerative cell proliferation for every cancer target site of chloroform in every strain of animal examined (International Programme on Chemical Safety 1994, Larson et al. 1994, 1995, 1996, Templin et al. 1995, 1996a, 1996b).

Chloroform caused a sustained cytolethal and regenerative cell proliferative response in the livers of female and male B6C3F1 mice under gavage dosing conditions similar to those that lead to cancer (National Cancer Institute 1976, Larson et al. 1994). Interestingly, similar daily doses of chloroform administered in drinking water did not induce hepatocellular damage, proliferation, or liver tumors (Larson et al. 1994, Jorgenson et al. 1985). This loss of carcinogenic activity is probably due to a slower dosing rate (the dose is fractionated because the animals drink two or three times during the day), resulting in a slower rate of formation of toxic metabolites that is not sufficient to kill cells (Larson et al. 1994). Complete loss of carcinogenic activity in a given target organ brought about by simply changing the vehicle and dose rate would not be expected of a mutagenic carcinogen. In the drinking water study, mice were exposed chronically to massive amounts of chloroform. Were chloroform directly mutagenic, irreversible mutations would accumulate even if they were formed at a slower rate. Because chloroform is a carcinogen only at cytolethal doses, those mutational and promotional events involved in its carcinogenicity are most likely secondary to cytolethality and regenerative cell proliferation.

Correlations Between Induced Cell Proliferation and Cancer

Both mutagenicity and induced cell proliferation are important to the carcinogenic process (Butterworth and Slaga 1991). However, understanding of the relationships between induced cell proliferation and cancer is somewhat limited from the lack of a large database in which both endpoints have been measured in parallel.

Studies thus far indicate that target organ-, sex-, strain-, and species-specific susceptibility factors need to be considered in correlating induced proliferation to tumor formation. A high degree of organ specificity and sensitivity is also seen for cancer induced by radiation and genotoxic carcinogens (Fry and Storer 1987, Walker et al. 1990). Examples of induced cell proliferation without induced cancer cannot be used to dismiss the concept of induced cell proliferation as playing a role in carcinogenesis any more than examples of noncarcinogenic mutagens (Tennant et al. 1987) can be used to dismiss the concept of mutagenesis in the carcinogenic process. Different degrees and lengths of sustained cell proliferation are required to produce tumors in different target organs and species. For example, although chloroform induces both liver and kidney toxicity in male BDF1 and B6C3F1 mice, the tissue susceptibility to cancer differs between the strains. Male BDF1 mice are particularly sensitive to the nephrotoxic effects of chloroform and nephrotoxic doses eventually lead to kidney cancer in this strain (Templin et al. 1996a, Yamamoto et al. 1994). In contrast to BDF1 mice, B6C3F1 mice carry the hepatocarcinogen susceptibility genes (*Hcs*) (Drinkwater 1994) and hepatotoxic doses of chloroform eventually produce liver cancer rather than kidney cancer in this strain (Larson et al. 1994, NCI 1976). This illustrates the important principle that genetic background and target organ specificity greatly influence tumor outcome. Thus, induced toxicity and regenerative cell proliferation are necessary but not always sufficient conditions to induce cancer in a given target organ.

Correlations of carcinogenic activity with in vitro and in vivo genotoxicity assays often have taken the form of simplistic plus-minus versus carcinogen-noncarcinogen comparisons with disregard for bioassay conditions, target organ specificity, and quantitative dose-response relationships. The situation with induced cell proliferation is more complex, and quantitative dose-response curves are required to establish the relationships of interest. Conditions used in the bioassay should be reproduced as closely as possible. Changing the dose, route of administration, or even the vehicle used to deliver the compound can have dramatic effects on both cell proliferation and the resulting tumor response (Larson et al. 1994). Rigorous attention should be paid to factors of dosimetry and target organ specificity in relating cell proliferation with cancer.

A further complication is that some agents may be affecting the growth of preneoplastic lesions only. In those cases, longer-term studies are required to see such effects.

Measurement of Cell Proliferation

In selecting doses for cancer studies, the pattern of induced cell proliferation cannot be viewed in isolation. Rather, it is an important adjunct to other critical data such as target organ toxicity and animal health. It is valuable to know whether induced cell proliferation is due to regeneration after necrosis or to direct mitogenic stimulation of growth (Butterworth et al. 1995). A histologic evaluation of the target tissues often provides this information. For example, liver sections from chloroform-treated mice under bioassay conditions exhibit extensive necrosis. In contrast, livers from rats treated with the mitogen di(2-ethylhexyl) phthalate are substantially larger, but no necrosis is evident. Release of liver-associated enzymes (such as alanine aminotransferase) into the serum provides further evidence of hepatic cytolethality.

Two commonly used methods for assessing the extent of cell replication are the labeling index (LI) and mitotic index. Whereas the mitotic index is a more precise measure of cell replication rates, the LI is more easily measured because mitosis is a brief event and low numbers of mitotic figures are observed in tissues. The kinetics of cell loss, including programmed cell death, termed apoptosis, can be of value in gaining a more complete understanding of the growth effects of a chemical. Apoptosis occurs rapidly and is thus difficult to detect and quantify (Bursch et al. 1984).

Variables of concern when conducting cell proliferation studies include animal age, species, chemical dose, treatment protocol, and the time and length that the label is administered. Many factors, such as diet, animal age, species, and dosing regimen are capable of modifying chemically induced cell proliferation responses. In retrospectively correlating a chemically induced S-phase response with carcinogenic activity, it is important to choose the animal species, doses, dosing regimen, and experimental conditions that produced tumors in the rodent cancer bioassay. If induced cell proliferation is used to aid in selecting doses for a cancer study, it is imperative to measure induced cell proliferation in the 13-week (90-day) study normally conducted as a prelude to the cancer study. In this way, cell proliferation rates will have been collected in the same strain of animal, at about the same point in time, and under conditions used in that laboratory. Greater confidence can be ascribed to such data compared with cell-proliferation studies that attempt to recapitulate study conditions from years before.

Setting Bioassay Doses

Principles in the Use of Cell-Proliferation Data in Dose Selection

Gathering chemically induced cell-proliferation data as part of the 13-week study that precedes a lifetime rodent pathogenesis study provides valuable information to aid in the rational selection of both the high and low doses and help in the eventual interpretation of the final outcome. Because induced cell proliferation greatly enhances tumor formation for both the genotoxic and nongenotoxic carcinogens, the principles presented here apply to any chemical in question.

Knowledge of target organs is critical. In some cases, this may be known from previous experience with the chemical or by analogy to structurally similar compounds with known activities. Target organ specificity often can be obtained by histologic examination of tissues from shorter-term studies that precede the 13-week study.

Induced cell proliferation is one critical endpoint used in conjunction with other key data, such as the dose-response curves for induced histopathologic changes, in setting rational doses for long-term cancer studies in rodents. Distinguishing a cytotoxic/regenerative response from a mitogenic response is important. A regenerative response is associated with cytolethality and necrosis and is sustained for 3–13 weeks. Dose-response curves for induced cell proliferation should be gathered in the time frame from 3 to 13 weeks. The following critical information usually can be identified from such studies: 1) animal health and the point at which the animals exhibit a 10% decrement in body weight gain; 2) doses of chemical that do not induce regenerative cell proliferation in the target organ; 3) the inflection point where regenerative cell proliferation becomes evident; and 4) doses that clearly induce regenerative cell proliferation.

Induced cell proliferation is a necessary, but not always sufficient, condition for tumor induction. The degree and duration of induced regenerative cell proliferation that will lead to tumors varies between species and target organs. Previous information on such relationships, when available, becomes a useful reference. As a general rule, increasing cell turnover by a factor of 3 or more over the baseline represents a significant increase in cell turnover and is indicative of a toxic response.

Sustained regenerative cell proliferation may strongly enhance the carcinogenic process. Including one dose that yields significantly elevated regenerative cell proliferation increases the probability of detecting nongenotoxic or weakly mutagenic carcinogens. However, that dose must not compromise animal health, as determined by parameters such as a decrement of greater than 10% in body-weight gain.

The strong enhancing effect of proliferation on the carcinogenic process confounds the extrapolation of the cancer response to lower, nontoxic doses. Thus, little is gained by conducting a cancer study with more than one dose of the agent that induces a significant, sustained increase in regenerative cell proliferation (Swenberg and Maronpot 1991). Addition of lower doses, including one that does not induce detectable regenerative cell proliferation, allows comparison of the dose-response curves for toxicity and carcinogenicity and greatly facilitates interpretation of any carcinogenic response.

For a cytotoxic-regenerative response for the high dose, the lowest dose should be chosen that induces a significant sustained increase in cell proliferation. Intermediate doses should be chosen about midway and at the inflection point of the induced cell proliferation dose-response curve. For the low dose, a dose should be chosen that clearly does not induce regenerative cell proliferation. In this way, the shapes of the toxicity and tumor curves can be compared to aid in interpretation of the final results.

Examples with Chloroform

Chloroform serves as an excellent example for the use of cell-proliferation data in selecting doses because a substantial number of tumor and corresponding induced cell-proliferation data are available. Chloroform produced liver cancer in both sexes of the B6C3F1 mouse (NCI 1976), kidney cancer in male Osborne–Mendel rats (NCI 1976, Jorgenson et al. 1985), and kidney cancer in male BDF1 mice (Yamamoto et al. 1994); it did not induce cancer in male or female Fisher 344 (F344) rats in an inhalation bioassay (Yamamoto et al. 1994). Cell proliferation dose-response curves have been gathered in all these species under conditions that approximate the original bioassays (Larson et al. 1994, 1995, 1996, Templin et al. 1995, 1996a, 1996b). This rich data set not only helps explain why tumors were formed in select target organs but also illustrates how knowledge of induced regenerative cell proliferation might have been used in advance to select more rational doses for the cancer studies.

The first step in this process is to determine that the chloroform-induced proliferative response observed in the liver and kidney is due to regenerative growth after a toxic insult. Evidence is strong that chloroform is acting through a nongenotoxic-cytotoxic mode of action in both the liver and kidney (International Programme on Chemical Safety 1994). Chloroform produces necrosis and histologic evidence of damage in both target tissues.

Table 1. Gavage administration of chloroform for 3 weeks in female B6C3F1 mice (Larson et al. 1994)

Dose (mg/kg/day)	Body weight vs. controls (%)	LI	Liver tumor outcome (%) (NCI 1976)
0	100	1.8 ± 0.7	0
3	105	1.3 ± 0.5	
10	100	1.9 ± 1.2	
34	110	2.7 ± 2.2	
90	111	2.7 ± 0.8*	
238[a]	106	11.0 ± 3.4*	80
477[b]	70	16.8 ± 3.4*	95

*Statistically increased from control group (Williams test, $p < 0.05$).
[a]One-half MTD.
[b]MTD.

The data in Table 1 illustrate the problem of selecting doses for cancer studies without knowledge of the occurrence of a strong cytolethal-regenerative response in a target organ (in this case, the liver). Chloroform produced liver cancer in the female mouse at both the MTD and one-half the MTD. However, there was also extensive liver necrosis and regenerative cell proliferation occurring at both doses that were probably responsible for driving tumor formation. Because proliferation is such a strong enhancer in the process of tumor formation, it is not possible to extrapolate from these doses to probable effects at the low doses associated with normal environmental levels of chloroform that do not induce toxicity or regenerative cell proliferation. Thus, nothing was gained by having two doses in the cytotoxic range, and much was lost by not knowing whether tumors were formed in the absence of the cytotoxic-regenerative response.

Using these cell proliferation data (Table 1) and the criteria noted above, more appropriate doses for the cancer study would be as follows:

High dose:	238 mg/kg/day
Intermediate dose:	90 mg/kg/day
Low dose:	10 mg/kg/day

Table 2. Administration of chloroform in drinking water of female B6C3F1 mice for 3 weeks (Larson et al. 1994)

Water conc. (ppm)	Body weight vs. controls (%)	LI	Liver tumor outcome (%) (Jorgenson et al. 1985)
0	100	2.7 ± 0.4	0
60	98	2.2 ± 1.4	
200	97	2.3 ± 1.2	4
400	96	2.6 ± 1.7	6
900	96	2.0 ± 0.8	0
1800	95	3.3 ± 2.2	2

Note: No labeling index value was statistically increased from the control group (Williams test, $p < 0.05$).

In this study of liver tumors, the group with the highest treatment received 1800 ppm of chloroform in the drinking water, which was near a saturated solution (Table 2). The animals receiving 1800 ppm (329 mg/kg/day) and 900 ppm (184 mg/kg/day) lost weight during the first week to a level below 80% of their initial body weight. This weight loss occurred because the animals refused to drink the chloroform-containing water and became dehydrated. In the bioassay study, 20% of the animals died from dehydration during the first week. However, body weights recovered during the second week as the animals became tolerant to the water containing chloroform.

Chloroform did not produce liver tumors in these animals even though they were receiving similar amounts of chloroform on a daily basis as noted above in the gavage study (Larson et al. 1994). This is probably because of the animals' ability to detoxify the small amounts of chloroform received at any one time from sips throughout the day. With the gavage study, the chloroform was given as a single bolus dose, which likely overwhelmed cellular defense mechanisms and resulted in liver necrosis. This lack of a tumor response by the drinking water route of administration is consistent with a lack of induced cell proliferation (Table 2).

Because there was no induced proliferation at any dose up to a saturated solution, the primary consideration in setting the doses for the bioassay for this data set would be the issue of animal health. Thus, all water concentrations of chloroform chosen with respect to cell proliferation were appropriate. The decision to use 1800 ppm, however, is questionable because of the initial dehydration that it produced in the animals.

Table 3. Inhalation exposure of female B6C3F1 mice to chloroform for 90 days (Larson et al. 1996)

Conc. in air (ppm)	Body weight vs. controls (%)	LI	Liver tumor outcome[a]
	Exposures: 7 days/week, 6 hours/day		
0	100	1.3 ± 1.8	
0.3	100	1.4 ± 1.0	
2	100	0.8 ± 0.3	
10	100	2.4 ± 1.5	
30	97	1.8 ± 1.4	
90	98	18.1 ± 5.9*	
	Exposures: 5 days/week, 6 hours/day		
10	107	0.8 ± 0.3	
90	97	7.1 ± 3.7*	

*Statistically increased from control group (Williams test, $p < 0.05$).
[a]Not yet known.

In the data set presented in Table 3, note the dramatic chloroform-induced toxicity in the liver as evidenced by cell turnover but without a significant loss in body-weight gain. One might have been tempted to use even higher atmospheric concentrations of chloroform because the decrease in body weight does not convey just how far one has moved into the toxic range for the liver. In this same study, there was no induced increase in the labeling index in the kidney.

Using these cell proliferation data (Table 3) and the criteria noted above, appropriate atmospheric concentrations for a cancer study with exposures of either 5 or 7 days/week would be as follows:

High dose:	90 ppm
Intermediate dose:	30 ppm
Low dose:	10 ppm

Table 4. Inhalation exposure of male BDF1 mice to chloroform for 4 days (Templin et al. 1996a)

Conc. in air (ppm)	Body weight vs. controls (%)	LI	Kidney tumor outcome (%) (Yamamoto et al. 1994)
	Exposures: 6 hours/day		
0	100	4.0 ± 1.1	0
0.3	93	3.3 ± 0.7	
5	94	2.6 ± 1.7	1
30	86	34.7 ± 13.7*	4
90	85	25.3 ± 8.8*	11

*Statistically increased from control group (Williams test, $p < 0.05$).

There are extenuating circumstances for the cancer data set in Table 4. Subjecting male BDF1 mice to atmospheres of 30 or 90 ppm of chloroform results in significant death with severe kidney pathology (Templin et al. 1996a). To keep the animals alive at these doses in the 2-year bioassay, the male mice in these groups were adapted by first exposing them to 2 ppm of chloroform for 2 weeks, then 10 ppm for two weeks, and then 30 ppm for two weeks (Yamamoto et al. 1994). Thus, it is questionable whether one can use these tumor data at all because of this unusual and artificial procedure.

Using these cell proliferation data (Table 4) and the criteria noted above, appropriate atmospheric concentrations for a cancer study for exposures of 5 days/week would be as follows:

High dose:	A dose between 5 and 30 ppm that results in no acute death or greater than 10% decrement in body weight gain
Intermediate dose:	5 ppm
Low dose:	1 ppm

In contrast to the males, the female BDF1 mice exposed to up to 90 ppm of chloroform exhibited no observed death, kidney toxicity, or regenerative cell proliferation or kidney tumors (Templin et al. 1996a, Yamamoto et al. 1994).

Table 5. Gavage single dose administration of chloroform to male Osborne-Mendel rats (Templin et al. 1995)

Dose (mg/kg/day)	Body weight vs. controls (%)	LI	Kidney tumor outcome (%) (NCI 1976)
0	100	0.4 ± 0.2	0
10	98	0.7 ± 0.2*	
90[a]	96	1.0 ± 0.4*	8
180[b]	95	1.7 ± 0.7*	24

*Statistically increased from control group (Williams test, $p < 0.05$).
[a]One-half MTD.
[b]MTD.

In this data set (Table 5) the relative response seen in the kidney is less than that seen with a cytotoxic insult in the liver. In this case, the dose-response curve is shallow. These data illustrate the problem of selecting doses for cancer studies without knowledge of the occurrence of a cytolethal regenerative response in a target organ. Chloroform produced kidney cancer in male Osborne–Mendel rats at both the MTD and one-half the MTD. However, necrosis and regenerative cell proliferation also occurred at both doses that were probably responsible for driving tumor formation. Because proliferation is such a strong enhancer in the process of tumor formation, it is not possible to extrapolate from these doses to probable effects at the low doses associated with normal environmental levels of chloroform. Little was gained by having two doses in the cytotoxic range, and much was lost by not knowing whether tumors were formed in the absence of the cytotoxic regenerative response.

Using these cell proliferation data (Table 5) and the criteria noted above, more appropriate doses for the cancer study would be as follows:

High dose:	180 mg/kg/day
Intermediate dose:	50 mg/kg/day
Low dose:	5 mg/kg/day

Table 6. Administration of chloroform in drinking water to male F344 rats for 3 weeks (Larson et al. 1995)

Water conc. (ppm)	Body weight vs. controls (%)	LI	Kidney cortex tumor outcome[a]
0	100	1.8 ± 0.2	
60	99	2.1 ± 0.5	
200	99	1.3 ± 0.4	
400	101	1.8 ± 0.3	
900	90	1.5 ± 0.8	
1800	81	1.8 ± 0.9	

Note: No labeling index value was statistically increased from control group.
[a]Not yet known.

In this study the group with the highest treatment received 1800 ppm of chloroform in the drinking water, which was near a saturated solution (Table 6). The animals in the group receiving 1800 ppm (106 mg/kg/day) actually lost weight during the course of this experiment. The animals in the group receiving 900 ppm (62 mg/kg/day) exhibited a decrement in body-weight gain of about 90% relative to the control animals. This value is about the cutoff used in selecting a highest dose for longer-term studies. Weight loss occurred because the animals refused to drink the chloroform-containing water and became dehydrated. Unlike the drinking water study in mice, water consumption remained depressed, and the rats did not become tolerant to the water containing chloroform.

Similar observations were noted in the 2-year drinking water study with male Osborne–Mendel rats (Jorgenson et al. 1985). Those rats receiving 1800 ppm of chloroform in the drinking water found it unpalatable and drank only about 60% as much as the control group. Because restricted water intake results in decreased food intake, the nutritional status of the high-dose group was uncertain. Terminal body weights from the high-dose group were only about 75% that of control animals (Jorgenson et al. 1985).

Induced cell proliferation in the kidney was chosen as the critical response (Table 6), because previous studies have established this as the primary target organ in the male rat. In this experiment, no increase in induced cell proliferation was noted up to a saturated solution. Therefore, the critical considerations for dose selection are animal health and reduced body weight gain. Using these criteria, concentrations for chloroform in the drinking water for the male F344 rat would be as follows:

High dose:	900 ppm
Intermediate dose:	400 ppm
Low dose:	200 ppm

Table 7. Inhalation exposure of male F344 rats to choloroform for 90 days (Templin et al. 1996b)

Conc. in air (ppm)	Body weight vs. controls (%)	LI	Liver tumor outcome
	Exposures: 7 days/week, 6 hours/day		
0	100	0.4 ± 0.3	—[a]
2	100	0.4 ± 0.2	—[a]
10	96	0.4 ± 0.2	—[a]
30	95	0.3 ± 0.1	—[a]
90	91	0.6 ± 0.3	—[a]
300	71	10.3 ± 6.0*	—[a]
	Exposures: 5 days/week, 6 hours/day		
0			None[b]
10			None[b]
30	95	0.4 ± 0.3	None[b]
90	89	0.2 ± 0.2	None[b]
300	69	11.6 ± 6.7*	

*Statistically increased from control group (Williams test, $p < 0.05$).
[a]Not yet known.
[b]From Yamamoto et al. 1994.

Because the chloroform-induced toxic effects were stronger in the kidney (Table 8) than in the liver (Table 7), it is the kidney data that should be used in selecting appropriate doses for the male rats.

Table 8. Inhalation exposure of male F344 rats to chloroform for 90 days (Templin et al. 1996b)

Conc. in air (ppm)	Body weight vs. controls (%)	LI	Kidney cortex tumor outcome
	Exposures: 7 days/week, 6 hours/day		
0	100	1.6 ± 0.4	—[a]
2	100	1.7 ± 0.6	—[a]
10	96	1.2 ± 0.3	—[a]
30	95	3.7 ± 1.8*	—[a]
90	91	6.7 ± 1.0*	—[a]
300	71	15.1 ± 2.2*	—[a]
	Exposures: 5 days/week, 6 hours/day		
0			None[b]
10			None[b]
30	95	1.5 ± 0.4	None[b]
90	89	2.7 ± 1.2*	None[b]
300	69	11.2 ± 2.7*	

*Statistically increased from control group (Williams test, $p < 0.05$).
[a]Not yet known.
[b]From Yamamoto et al. 1994.

These data show that the kidney and not the liver is the more-sensitive target organ for setting doses for longer-term studies. The exposure concentration of 300 ppm at either 5 or 7 days/week has too strong an adverse effect on animal health and body-weight gain to be used in longer-term studies.

Using these cell proliferation data (Table 8) and the criteria noted above, appropriate atmospheric concentrations for a cancer study with exposures of either 5 or 7 days/week would be as follows:

High dose:	90 ppm
Intermediate dose:	30 ppm
Low dose:	10 ppm

Whereas one might expect a tumor response in the kidneys of male rats exposed to 90 ppm of chloroform 7 days/week, that response probably would not be seen with a 90-ppm regimen for 5 days/week, based on the premise that induced cell proliferation might drive tumor formation in the male rat kidney (Table 8). In fact, the inhalation study of Yamamoto et al. (1994) was conducted for 5 days/week and no visible kidney tumors were induced at 90 ppm.

Conclusions

Chemically induced cell proliferation is an important consideration in setting doses for cancer studies for genotoxic as well as nongenotoxic carcinogens. The first step in utilizing such information is to distinguish between a mitogenic and a cytotoxic regenerative response. For cytotoxicants, because sustained regenerative cell proliferation may strongly enhance the carcinogenic process, including one dose that yields significantly elevated regenerative cell proliferation, the probability of detecting nongenotoxic or weakly mutagenic carcinogens is increased. However, that dose must not compromise animal health, as determined by a number of parameters such as a decrement of greater than 10% in body-weight gain or severe organ dysfunction or pathologic changes. Increased regenerative cell proliferation, in itself, serves as a clear indicator of compromised animal health. The same enhancing effect of induced proliferation on the carcinogenic process also prevents extrapolation of the cancer response to lower, nontoxic doses. Thus, little is gained by conducting a cancer study with more than one dose of the agent that induces a significant, sustained increase in regenerative cell proliferation (Swenberg and Maronpot 1991). Addition of lower doses that do not induce regenerative cell proliferation allows comparison of the toxicity and carcinogenicity dose-response curves and greatly facilitates interpretation of any carcinogenic response. The extensive data sets for chloroform-induced cell proliferation discussed in this section serve as an example of the value of such information in selection of doses for cancer studies for such cytotoxic agents.

The transient increase in cell proliferation seen with mitogens often is associated with additive hyperplasia as the target organ is stimulated to increase and maintain a larger size with continued dosing of the chemical. Because the period of increased proliferation is so brief, it is less clear that this pattern of cell proliferation is as actively involved in driving tumor formation as is a sustained regenerative response. In this case, including more than one dose that induces this mitogenic response may be appropriate. However, because stimulation of mitogenic activity may be driving tumor formation by providing a selective growth advantage to precancerous cells, it remains important to include at least one dose at which detectable mitogenic activity is not present to aid in the interpretation of results from the cancer study. For a mitogenic response, doses should be chosen based on criteria of altered animal health and no more than a 10% decrement in body-weight gain.

DOSE SELECTION FOR SODIUM SACCHARIN AS INFLUENCED BY CELL PROLIFERATION[3]

Sodium saccharin illustrates the difficulties of evaluating the carcinogenicity of a substance that is quite nontoxic and is nongenotoxic. Very high doses can be administered in the diet or drinking water of rodents with impunity, easily attaining levels of 5% of the diet without reaching a MTD defined by a decrease in body weight of 10% or more (International Agency for Research on Cancer 1980, Ellwein and Cohen 1990). By light microscopy, there are no obvious toxic effects on any tissues at these doses; in fact, there is actually a decrease in the nephropathy of male rats, resulting in a prolongation of life compared to untreated controls (IARC 1980, Ellwein and Cohen 1990, Schoenig et al. 1985). A further difficulty with sodium saccharin is its lack of carcinogenicity in the standard 2-year bioassay beginning at 7–8 weeks of age (IARC 1980, Ellwein and Cohen 1990). Carcinogenicity appears only when administration begins at an earlier age, for example, as in a two-generation protocol including feeding to the F_0 generation before mating, then to the dam during pregnancy and lactation, and continuing administration to the offspring of the F_0 generation in the diet for the remainder of its life span.

If sodium saccharin were being addressed today in standard fashion without any prior clues about its carcinogenicity, it would be hard to select doses based on any clues arising from a subchronic (13 week) assay. However, as early as 1970 (IARC 1980, Bryan et al. 1970), there was some evidence that sodium saccharin had an effect on the lower urinary tract epithelium, the urothelium. This provided some direction for dose selection. However, the mainstay of even the two-generation bioassays in rats with sodium saccharin have relied on 5% as an arbitrary maximum dose, whether toxicity was observed or not (IARC 1980, Ellwein and Cohen 1990, Schoenig et al 1985). Results have been positive in rats at this dose, particularly males, although higher doses have been used (IARC 1980, Ellwein and Cohen 1990, Schoenig et al. 1985). However, no effects are observed on the urothelium in mice at a dietary dose of 5% or even as high as 7.5%, a dose considerably higher, on a mg/kg basis, than that used in rats (IARC 1980, Ellwein and Cohen 1990, Frederick et al. 1989). In retrospect, it is possible to identify doses that not only are helpful in evaluating the carcinogenicity of sodium saccharin but also are useful in further defining mechanistic information in a correlative fashion.

The various two-generation bioassays with sodium saccharin in rats have examined a wide range of doses (IARC 1980, Ellwein and Cohen 1990, Schoenig et al. 1985), as listed in Table 9. Positive results have been obtained in male rats relatively consistently at a dose level of 5% of the diet, whereas doses of 1% and lower have been consistently negative. The study by Schoenig et al.

---

[3] Contributed by Samuel M. Cohen.

(1985) examined the dose response in detail; their experimental design used an unbalanced group size, with much larger groups than ordinarily are used in bioassays (350 rats in the control group and 700 in the 1% sodium saccharin group). Doses from 1% to 7.5% of the diet were tested, with a clearly defined, statistical no-effect level at 1% of the diet and a minimal, but statistically significant effect at 3% of the diet (based on the original histopathology). Evaluation of sodium saccharin in one-generation studies but administered after a brief exposure to a carcinogen, such as *N*-[4-(5-nitro-2-furyl)-2-thiazolyl] formamide (IARC 1980, Ellwein and Cohen 1990), *N*-butyl-*N*-(4-hydroxybutyl)nitrosamine (Nakanishi et al. 1980), *N*-methyl-*N*-nitrosourea (IARC 1980, Ellwein and Cohen 1990, West et al. 1986), or cyclophosphamide (Cohen et al. 1982) or after freeze ulceration (Cohen et al. 1982, Hasegawa et al. 1985) also generally showed positive results at a dose level of 5% of the diet. Positive results in such studies also have been observed at 2.5% and 3% of the diet, but consistently negative results are observed at a dose of 1%, mimicking carcinogenicity results of two-generation bioassays (Nakanishi et al. 1980, Cohen et al. 1991).

Because sodium saccharin is nongenotoxic toward the target tissue, the rat urothelial carcinogenicity must arise from increased cell proliferation (Ellwein and Cohen 1990, Cohen and Ellwein 1990, Ellwein and Cohen 1988). Two-generation or one-generation short-term studies, with exposures as brief as 1 week or as long as 18 weeks, showed increased proliferation with sodium saccharin in the male rat bladder epithelium, with a clear dose response (Ellwein and Cohen 1990, Fukushima and Cohen 1980, Murasaki and Cohen 1981, Cohen et al. 1990, Garland et al. 1991, and unpublished observations). The dose of 5% of the diet consistently produced increased urothelial proliferation as did higher doses, but lower doses have produced variable responses. Nevertheless, it appears that doses of 2.5% or 3% are the lowest doses at which a positive effect was observed, whereas doses of 1% and below were without effect (IARC 1980, Bryan et al. 1970, Garland et al. 1991, unpublished observations), similar to the dose response in carcinogenesis bioassays. This has been the case even when the hyperplastic and proliferative effects are examined by extremely sensitive measures, including labeling indices and observation of the bladder surface by scanning electron microscopy (Cohen et al. 1990). Thus, if one were preparing to evaluate bladder carcinogenicity of sodium saccharin, one could design a relatively short-term study, certainly within the usual 13 weeks of subchronic study, evaluating the dose response of cell proliferation with doses above and below 2.5% of the diet, which appears to be the lowest effective dose for sodium saccharin even in the most susceptible species/sex, the male rat. There has been a close correlation between doses at which there is a positive effect with respect to increased cell proliferation and a positive effect in carcinogenicity studies.

Dose-response information for sodium saccharin subsequently has been utilized to focus on various mechanistic considerations in attempting to determine the cause of increased urothelial proliferation. The increased proliferation of the urothelium appears to be due to a cytotoxic effect on the superficial cells, the effect again present at 2.5% or 3% of the diet and higher but not at 1% or lower (Fukushima and Cohen 1980, Murasaki and Cohen 1981, Cohen et al. 1990). Extensive biochemical and nutritional effects have been examined in a dose-response manner and have produced a distinction between a positive effect at a dose of 3% and above with no response at a dose of 1% of the diet (Garland et al. 1991). More recently, the likely cause of the cytotoxicity has been identified as the formation of an amorphous precipitate in the urine of rats administered high doses of sodium saccharin. A variety of manipulations of the diet can alter the formation of this precipitate, which correlates closely with the production of a hyperplastic and tumorigenic response (Ellwein and Cohen 1990, Cohen et al. 1995). Thus, administration of sodium saccharin as 3% of the diet or higher yields production of this amorphous precipitate, whereas administration as 1% of the diet is without effect, with respect to either formation of the precipitate or production of hyperplasia (Cohen et al. 1995, unpublished observations). Similarly, any treatment that inhibits the formation of the amorphous precipitate, such as administration with ammonium chloride to produce an acidic urine, also inhibits the production of hyperplasia (Ellwein and Cohen 1990).

The focus of all of these studies, whether specific mechanistic evaluations, production of hyperplasia, or production of tumors, utilizes doses above and below a minimally effective level to establish as strong a correlation as possible between the variables. For short-term studies, several doses can be used, and this is most helpful in defining as closely as possible the necessary correlations. For long-term, carcinogenicity bioassays, fewer doses are feasible but, again, the emphasis should be on defining doses above and below a minimally effective dose as predicted from short-term assays. It is in this way that cell proliferation data can be utilized for establishing doses for a chronic bioassay (Cohen and Ellwein 1990, Cohen and Ellwein 1991, Cohen and Ellwein 1992). A minimally effective dose for increased cell proliferation can be defined in a 13-week subchronic bioassay, with doses above and below this minimally effective dose being selected for the chronic 2-year bioassay. This, of course, assumes that one can identify increased proliferation in potential target tissues for carcinogenicity. Use of such cell proliferation data could help in addressing the difficulties of trying to define and utilize a MTD or various fractions thereof. Rather than routinely using the MTD, one-half the MTD, and one-fourth the MTD, it is necessary to define doses relative to a marker of cell proliferation, with doses selected above and below a minimally effective dose in a subchronic study.

Table 9. Urinary bladder carcinogenicity of sodium saccharin in male F_1 generation rats in two-generation studies

Study	Dose (% of diet)	No. of rats	No. of rats with bladder cancer
Tisdel et al[a]	0	12	0
	0.05	10	0
	0.5	11	0
	5	15	7 (47)
Taylor and Friedman[a]	0	29	0
	0.01	28	0
	0.1	31	0
	1.0	30	0
	5.0	21	0
	7.5	23	4 (17)
Arnold et al[a]	0	42	0
	5	45	12 (27)
Schoenig et al (1985)	0	324	0
	1.0	658	1 (0.2)
	3.0	472	4 (0.8)
	4.0	189	8 (4.2)
	5.0	120	11 (9.2)
	6.25	120	8 (6.7)
	7.5	118	19 (16.1)

[a]Summarized in Bryan et al. (1970).

Applying these principles to sodium saccharin, doses for a long-term two-generation bioassay could be chosen based on the results of a short-term cell proliferation study. Because there is little toxicity, the highest dose would be 5% of the diet. The most appropriate intermediate dose would be 2.5% of the diet, because it is the lowest effective dose that produces an increase in urothelial proliferation. The lowest dose would be 1% of the diet, because it is without effect in producing increased cell proliferation. This would be more appropriate than 1.25% of the diet (one-fourth of the MTD), because it is clearly negative and no data exist for the 1.25% dose. It is essential to have at least one dose clearly below the dose required to produce an effect in short-term screening studies—in this case, cell proliferation.

The issues described above address only the issue of dose selection for a chronic bioassay in rodents, and for sodium saccharin this pertains only to rats. Regardless of doses selected, it must be kept in mind that the bioassay is merely a screen for detecting human carcinogens. If positive in the bioassay, other information is needed for dose and species extrapolation. Carcinogenesis might be strictly a high-dose phenomenon, as is the case with sodium saccharin. An evaluation of human exposure then is of critical importance. The 1% dietary level of sodium saccharin in rats is more than 100 times the level of human exposure. Also, carcinogenesis in rodents might be species specific and not pertinent to humans based on mechanistic considerations, such as chemicals producing α_{2U}-globulin-related kidney tumors in male rats. Sodium and potassium salts (such as sodium saccharin) produce bladder tumors in rats, which appear not only to be restricted to high doses but also to be species specific (only the rat).

DOSE SELECTION: METABOLIC SATURATION[4]

Introduction

It is well known that the toxicity of many compounds is determined by metabolically based transformation and elimination processes. Metabolic processes may convert relatively nontoxic parent compounds to metabolites that are ultimately responsible for expression of toxicity. Cellular metabolic events also may transform toxicologically active parent compounds or their metabolites to toxicologically inactive products, thus contributing directly to detoxification of the chemical. Similarly, detoxification of some chemicals or their active metabolites is determined directly by metabolic processes such as active transport mechanisms that facilitate elimination of toxicants from the body. Because metabolically based activation, detoxification, and elimination systems responsible for modulating toxicity are by definition capacity limited, they are potentially subject to metabolic saturation under conditions of high-dose compound administration.

Saturation of critical metabolic transformation or elimination processes often is concurrently associated with nonlinear expression of toxicity over the range of doses evaluated in chronic animal bioassays. Use of saturating doses can create scenarios in which abnormally high, dose-dependent tissue concentrations of a toxicant or its toxic metabolite(s) are uniquely attained in target tissues. Thus, as presented in several representative examples below, high-dose specific toxicity can be attributed to toxic mechanisms that are operative only under conditions of saturated metabolism or elimination.

Information describing the toxicokinetic behavior of test compounds over the range of test doses applied in chronic bioassays can provide extremely valuable insights into the relevance of nonlinear, high-dose-associated animal toxicity responses to potential human risk. In addition, if appropriately designed toxicokinetic and metabolic information can be obtained before initiation of chronic bioassays, such data can be criteria for dose selection. The concepts described above perhaps can be best visualized by the provision of several illustrative examples.

Vinyl Chloride

Chronic inhalation studies with vinyl chloride in rats have demonstrated that the incidence of hepatic angiosarcomas increased at exposure concentrations of 50, 250, 500, and 2500 ppm (Maltoni and Lefemine 1975). However, the incidence of angiosarcomas increased less than 2-fold as the exposure

[4] Contributed by James Bus.

concentration increased 5-fold from 500 to 2500 ppm. In addition, the incidence of angiosarcomas was essentially equal in rats exposed to vinyl chloride concentrations of 2500, 6000, and 10,000 ppm. A plausible explanation for this plateau in tumorigenic response rests in the fundamental observation that both the genotoxicity and liver toxicity of vinyl chloride is mediated through metabolism to a reactive metabolite (Gehring et al. 1978). Importantly, additional metabolism studies have shown that exposure-limited formation of a reactive metabolite at these higher exposures can be attributed to saturation of the mixed-function oxidase enzyme responsible for generation of the toxic metabolite (Gehring et al. 1978).

Experimental evidence identifying the dose at which metabolic saturation has been achieved can be obtained from dose-dependent comparisons of several toxicokinetic parameters. In the case of vinyl chloride, a volatile hydrocarbon, Gehring et al. (1977) reported that dose-disproportionate changes in the exhalation of the parent compound occurred between inhalation exposures of 10 and 1000 ppm. Further studies demonstrated that nonlinear changes in total nonvolatile radioactivity remaining in the carcass immediately after termination of a 6-hour inhalation exposure (regarded as a good indicator of total vinyl chloride metabolism) occurred between exposure concentrations of 500 and 1000 ppm (Gehring et al. 1978). These relatively straightforward observations can be used to estimate that metabolic saturation occurs between 500 and 1000 ppm for 6-hour exposure regimens. This estimate agrees remarkably well with the exposure concentrations at which the tumorigenic response of vinyl chloride plateaued.

Toxicokinetic data such as that described above, if obtained before the bioassay is designed, could have provided a principle-based argument for limiting the top dose in the vinyl chloride bioassay to between 500 and 1000 ppm. In the face of a lack of a priori knowledge of the chronic bioassay outcome, selection of top bioassay exposures greater than these concentrations would clearly run the risk of producing toxicity that might be entirely attributable to disproportionate increases in tissue concentrations of the parent compound. Although this did not turn out to be the case for vinyl chloride, investigators nonetheless could have reasonably assumed that such an accumulation of parent compound might produce toxicity capable of compromising long-term survival of the animals. In addition, and of equal importance when compounds with toxicokinetic behavior similar to that of vinyl chloride are used, if known human exposures are significantly less than the level at which metabolic saturation occurs, then the unique high-dose-dependent toxicity observed above metabolic saturation conditions would likely be irrelevant for human risk assessment. However, if human exposure concentrations are known to approach or exceed the demonstrated metabolic saturation concentration, the highest animal bioassay dose selected should be above the identified saturation point.

Although the example of vinyl chloride is one in which expression of toxicity is actually limited by metabolic saturation issues, perhaps the more common scenario is that in which toxicity develops only when a critical detoxification pathway, rather than bioactivation pathways, is saturated under high-dose conditions. Experiences with the chronic bioassays of two chemicals, *o*-phenylphenol (OPP) and methylene chloride, illustrate this issue.

o-Phenylphenol

Rats fed high concentrations of OPP in the diet (1–4%) developed malignant bladder tumors, whereas dietary doses of 0.5% or less produced no evidence of bladder tumors (Hiraga and Fujii 1981). The steep nature of the tumorigenic response suggested that a critical metabolic detoxification pathway was likely saturated under high-dose-only conditions (>1% OPP in the diet), resulting in an inability of target cells to further hold in check the tissue-damaging potential of an OPP-derived reactive metabolite. Metabolism studies conducted by Reitz et al. (1983, 1984) demonstrated that OPP was completely metabolized to sulfate and glucuronide conjugates at low-dose exposures. However, at the bioassay tumorigenic doses, increasing amounts of OPP escaped sulfate/glucuronide conjugation and were subject to mixed function oxidase metabolism to reactive quinone metabolites capable of covalently binding to tissue macromolecules. Importantly, tissue covalent binding was nonlinear with dose and increased disproportionately in tissues, including bladder, at the metabolically saturating carcinogenic doses.

The covalent binding of OPP in bladder tissue correlated with histopathologic evidence of tissue damage as well as stimulation of cellular DNA synthesis (Reitz et al. 1984). Although high-dose-associated macromolecular covalent binding of OPP was detectable in bladder epithelial cells, actual binding of OPP-derived metabolite to DNA was not observed, consistent with the demonstrated lack of OPP genotoxicity. Thus, the carcinogenic activity of OPP appeared to be secondary to cytotoxic responses that occur only under conditions of metabolic saturation of key detoxification pathways.

In the example of OPP, the profiling of urinary metabolites over a range of doses provided clear evidence of high-dose-dependent metabolic saturation. Rats receiving oral doses of 50 mg/kg or less excreted only the sulfate and glucuronide conjugates of OPP in urine. However, when rats were dosed with OPP at 500 mg/kg, a third metabolite identified as the sulfate or glucuronide conjugate of the likely reactive quinone metabolite of OPP was detected in urine at significant concentrations. Consistent with these observations, additional evidence of high-dose-specific metabolic saturation was provided from in vivo macromolecular binding studies in which covalent binding in bladder, liver, and kidney was investigated (Rao et al. 1985). Tissue binding was linear at doses up to 100 mg/kg, whereas dramatic nonlinearities in binding were apparent at doses of 200 and 500 mg/kg. Because doses of 200 to 500 mg/kg are significantly above the potential human exposures to OPP, such data could have provided a strong toxicokinetic rationale for limiting the top dose in the animal bioassay to no more than 100 mg/kg/day. Importantly, such a dose strategy would have avoided introduction of the likely irrelevant issue of high-dose-specific rodent bladder tumors into the final human risk assessment.

Methylene Chloride

The example of methylene chloride is differentiated from that of OPP in that it describes a situation in which the ultimate metabolic toxification pathway is not fully functional until an alternative nontoxic metabolic detoxification pathway operating at low exposure doses is overwhelmed (saturated). A series of rodent bioassays provided evidence that methylene chloride tumorigenicity was distinctly high-dose specific. A drinking water study with doses up to 250 mg/kg/day did not produce any evidence of a dose-related increase in tumors in either B6C3F1 mice or F344 rats (Serota et al. 1984). However, the incidence of benign and malignant liver and lung tumors was increased in B6C3F1 mice after chronic inhalation exposure to methylene chloride at 2000 or 4000 ppm, while only benign tumors were noted in similarly exposed F344 rats (NTP 1985). These species-specific and dose-dependent findings suggested that alterations in metabolism might account for the varied tumorigenic responses.

A combination of in vitro and in vivo metabolism studies has led to definition of two distinctly different competing and dose- dependent metabolic pathways for methylene chloride (Ahmed and Anders 1978, Kubic et al. 1974). In a series of studies designed to construct a physiologically based pharmacokinetic (PB-PK) model for methylene chloride (Anderson et al. 1987, Reitz et al. 1988, 1989), the two competing metabolic pathways available for metabolism, cytochrome P450-based oxidation and glutathione transferase-mediated conjugation, were found to have clearly different metabolic capacities. The cytochrome P450-mediated pathway was identified as high affinity but low capacity in its ability to metabolize methylene chloride. In contrast, the glutathione transferase-mediated pathway was determined to be a low-affinity but high-capacity process. The metabolic implications of these findings were that the oxidative pathway predominated under low methylene chloride exposure conditions and the glutathione pathway became increasingly dominant at higher exposures.

A series of biochemical and genetic toxicity studies have supported the contention that the glutathione transferase pathway leads to formation of genotoxic and cytotoxic metabolites. The oxidative pathway, however, likely results in production of metabolites with diminished toxicity potential (summarized in Reitz et al. 1989). The PB-PK model clearly predicts that the oxidative detoxification pathway would not be saturated at the dose levels administered in the chronic oral bioassay, thus limiting the potential formation of a likely carcinogenic metabolite(s). This prediction is consistent with the lack of tumorigenic response in the drinking water study.

In contrast, the PB-PK model predicts that tissue concentrations arising from the 2000-ppm or the 4000-ppm inhalation exposures would be sufficient to saturate the capabilities of the oxidative pathway and that the glutathione transferase pathway would be a significant metabolic route under these exposure conditions. The glutathione transferase pathway would not be expected to contribute significantly to methylene chloride metabolism at low tissue concentrations because of its low affinity for the chemical substrate. Similar to the oral dose scenario, the positive tumorigenic outcome of the inhalation study was entirely consistent with the predictions of the model.

Although it is unlikely that a PB-PK model would be developed before a chronic bioassay is designed, the model nonetheless illustrates the potential consequences of selecting top doses for rodent cancer bioassays that bear no relationship to environmental human exposures. The drinking water assay was designed to assess the human health implications of very low environmental exposures to methylene chloride. Thus, the selection of a top dose of 250 mg/kg/day represented a very large differential between the animal bioassay top dose and potential human environmental exposures. If the top dose of the oral study had been pushed even higher, the PB-PK model suggests that a positive tumorigenic response might have been obtained. However, because the model also predicts that the tumorigenic response would have been attributable to metabolic pathways that function only at high doses, the predictive value of such a finding for human risk assessment would have been questionable.

In a similar context, the inhalation bioassay was designed primarily to evaluate the potential hazard associated with occupational exposure to methylene chloride. The PB-PK model clearly demonstrated that both bioassay exposure concentrations selected, 2000 and 4000 ppm, saturated the critical low-level detoxification pathway. Thus, the inhalation bioassay as conducted failed to adequately assess a critical element of the risk-assessment process, the dose-response characterization.

Propylene Glycol Monomethyl Ether

The examples of vinyl chloride, OPP, and methylene chloride represent situations in which metabolic information was used to provide perspective to the interpretation of existing chronic bioassays in animals. In fact, the design of the metabolism studies for these compounds was significantly facilitated by knowledge of the chronic bioassay response. This observation should not imply, however, that metabolic information cannot be used to effectively facilitate dose selection before initiation of a bioassay. Information gathered from both acute and subchronic toxicity studies, coupled with a focused-design metabolism study, may well provide the needed rationale for appropriate dose selection in chronic bioassays. The design of a chronic rodent bioassay for propylene glycol monomethyl ether (PGME) (Corley 1994) illustrates an approach to dose selection that linked acute and subchronic toxicity findings with metabolism information to facilitate bioassay dose selection.

The acute inhalation exposure toxicity of PGME was characterized by mortality in mice exposed to greater than 6000 ppm of PGME; severe sedation accompanied these exposures in both mice and rats. PGME-induced sedation also was apparent in mice and rats receiving a single acute exposure of 3000 ppm. However, the sedation effect was transient and resolved after several 6-hour/day exposures. Resolution of the sedation response was accompanied by increased liver weights in both rats and mice. Single or repeated exposures to PGME at 300 and 1000 ppm did not cause any treatment-related effects, including sedation. Importantly, 90-day toxicity studies conducted in mice and rats at a top exposure concentration of 3000 ppm (Landry et al. 1983, Corley 1994) also found no evidence of treatment-related effects other than transient central nervous system depression during the first several days of exposure, increased liver weights in both mice and rats, and mild changes in renal histopathology in male rats (shown to be an α_{2u}-globulin nephropathy).

Metabolism studies in rats and mice provided important insight into the possibility that the high-dose-associated sedation effects of PGME, and their resolution by using repeated dose protocols, was likely due to initial saturation and subsequent metabolic adaptation of the key metabolic step involved in detoxification of PGME. A primary metabolic pathway for PGME involved oxidative O-demethylation to propylene glycol (Miller et al. 1983). A subsequent metabolism study in rats (Morgott and Nolan 1987) demonstrated that the O-demethylation of PGME was likely subject to metabolic saturation at exposure concentrations exceeding 1500 ppm, as evidenced by a linear increase in blood propylene glycol concentration after single 6-hour inhalation exposures to PGME at 750 and 1500 ppm and no further increase in blood propylene glycol after a 3000-ppm exposure. Evidence that metabolic adaptation likely accounted for resolution of the sedation response was supported by the observation that PGME blood concentrations at the end of a 6-hour exposure were reduced approximately 45% in rats receiving 10 repeated 6-hour/day exposures relative to those receiving a single exposure. In addition, the reduction in blood PGME concentration was accompanied by evidence of adaptive enzyme induction characterized by increased liver cytochrome P450 content and aniline hydroxylase and *p*-nitroanisole O-demethylase activities.

Increased liver oxidative metabolic enzyme activity also was noted in mice repeatedly exposed to 3000 ppm of PGME (Corley 1994).

Given the lack of body-weight effects and significant treatment-related histopathologic effects, consideration of the standard toxicity data from the 90-day PGME studies alone did not provide a compelling rationale for limitation of the top exposure concentration to 3000 ppm for the chronic bioassay. However, clear evidence from pharmacokinetic studies that a 3000-ppm exposure approached or even likely exceeded saturation of the metabolic pathway accountable for detoxifying the sedative activity of the parent PGME argued for limitation of the top dose to no greater than 3000 ppm. In addition, taken by themselves, the acute and subchronic studies suggested that animals not only might survive but also might exhibit minimal toxicity to repeated PGME exposures above 3000 ppm but below 6000 ppm. However, the metabolic enzyme studies provided the clear warning that the long-term health status and survival of animals exposed to concentrations above 3000 ppm was likely dependent on maintenance of an elevated compensatory metabolism state. Indeed, even at the top bioassay concentration of 3000 ppm, a gradual return of sedation after 52 weeks of exposure correlated with a return of oxidative enzyme activity to near control levels (Corley 1994). Thus, the example of PGME illustrates that responses such as metabolic adaptation may be important factors in addition to pharmacokinetic studies for considerations of top-dose selection for chronic bioassays.

REFERENCES

Ahmed AE, Anders MW (1978) Metabolism of dihalomethanes to formaldehyde and inorganic halide. I. In vitro studies. Drug Metab Dispos 4:357–361

Allegretta M, Nicklas JA, Siram S, Albertini RJ (1990) T cells responsive to myelin basic protein in patients with multiple sclerosis. Science 247:718–721

Ames BN, Gold LS (1990) Too many rodent carcinogens. Science 249:970–971

Andersen ME, Clewell HJ, Gargas ML, et al (1987) Physiologically based pharmacokinetics and the risk assessment for methylene chloride. Toxicol Appl Pharmacol 87:185–205

Anon (1990a) Bioassay of limonene for rodent carcinogenicity.
NTP report RT 347. National Institutes of Health, Bethesda, MD

Anon (1990b) Bioassay of glycidol for rodent carcinogenicity.
NTP report TR 374. National Institutes of Health, Bethesda, MD

Anon (1993a) Toxicology and carcinogenesis studies of benzyl acetate. NTP Technical Report 431. National Institutes of Health, Bethesda, MD

Anon (1993b) Toxicology and carcinogenesis studies of acetaminophen in

F344/N rats and B6C3F1 mice (feed studies): US National Toxicology Program, TR 394. National Institutes of Health, Bethesda, MD

Apostolou A (1990) Relevance of maximum tolerated dose to human carcinogenic risk. Reg Toxicol Pharmacol 11:68–80

Argyris TS (1980) Tumor promotion by abrasion induced epidermal hyperplasia in the skin of mice. J Invest Dermatol 75:360–362

Argyris TS (1989) Epidermal tumor promotion by damage in the skin of mice. In Slaga TJ (ed), Skin Carcinogenesis: Mechanisms and Human Relevance. Alan R. Liss, New York, pp 63–80

Ashby J (1994a) Two million rodent carcinogens? The role of SAR and QSAR in their detection. Mut Res 30.5:3–13

Ashby J (1994b) Benzyl acetate: from mutagenic carcinogen to non-mutagenic noncarcinogen in 7 years? Mut Res 30.6:107–109

Ashby J, Morrod RS (1991) Detection of human carcinogens. Nature 352:185–186

Ashby J, Tennant RW (1994) Prediction of rodent carcinogenicity for 44 chemicals results. Mutagenesis 9:7–15

Ashby J, Tinwell H (1994) Comparative activity of human carcinogens and NTP rodent carcinogens in the mouse bone marrow micronucleus assay. Environ Health Perspect, in press.

Bailey A, Saliba D, Miller DM (1989) A marked increase in sensitivity to carcinogenesis is associated with induced protooncogene expression without DNA synthesis. Proc Am Assoc Cancer Res 30:183

Bailey A, Sanchez JD, Rigsby D, Roesel J, Alvarez R, Rodu B, Miller DM (1990) Stimulation of renal and hepatic c-myc and c-Ha-ras expression by unilateral nephrectomy. Oncogene Res 5:287–293

Belinsky SA, Walker VE, Maronpot RR, Swenberg JA, Anderson MW (1987) Molecular dosimetry of DNA adduct formation and cell toxicity in rat nasal mucosa following exposure to the tobacco specific nitrosamine 4-(N-methyl-N-nitroamino)-1-(3-pyridyl)-1-butanone and their relationship to induction of neoplasia. Cancer Res 47:6058–6065

Borghoff SJ, Short BG, Swenberg JA (1990) Biochemical mechanisms and pathobiology of α_{2u}-globulin nephropathy. Annu Rev Pharmacol Toxicol 30:349–367

Braun L, Mead JE, Panzica M, Mikumo R, Bell GI, Fausto N (1988) Transforming growth factor beta mRNA increases during liver regeneration: a possible paracrine mechanism of growth regulation. Proc Natl Acad Sci 85:1539–1543

Bryan GT, Erturk E, Yoshida O (1970) Production of urinary bladder carcinomas in mice by sodium saccharin. Science 168:1238–1240

Bursch W, Lauer B, Timmermann-Trosiner I, et al (1984) Controlled death (apoptosis) of normal and putative preneoplastic cells in rat liver following withdrawal of tumor promoters. Carcinogenesis 5:453–458

Butterworth B (1990) Consideration of both genotoxic and non-genotoxic mechanisms in predicting carcinogenic potential. Mut Res 239:117–132

Butterworth BE, Conolly RB, Morgan KT (1995) A strategy for establishing mode of action of chemical carcinogens as a guide for approaches to risk assessments. Cancer Letters 93:129–146

Butterworth BE, Slaga TJ, eds (1991) Chemically Induced Cell Proliferation: Implications for Risk Assessment. Progress in Clinical and Biological Research, Vol. 369. Wiley-Liss, New York.

Casanova M, Deyo D, Heck H (1989) Covalent binding of inhaled formaldehyde to DNA in the nasal mucosa of Fischer 344 rats: Analysis of formaldehyde and DNA by high-performance liquid chromatography and provisional pharmacokinetic interpretation. Fundam Appl Toxicol 12:397–417

Cattley RC, Popp JA (1989) Differences between the promoting activities of the peroxisome proliferator Wy-14,643 and phenobarbital in rat liver. Cancer Res 49:3246–3251

Cayama E, Tsuda H, Sarma DSR, Farber E (1978) Initiation of chemical carcinogenesis requires cell proliferation. Nature 275:60–62

Cohen SM, Cano M, Garland EM, et al (1995) Urinary and urothelial effects of sodium salts in male rats. Carcinogenesis 16:343–348

Cohen SM, Ellwein LB (1990) Cell proliferation in carcinogenesis. Science 249:1007–1011

Cohen SM, Ellwein LB (1991) Genetic errors, cell proliferation, and carcinogenesis. Cancer Res 51:6493–6505

Cohen SM, Ellwein LB (1992) Risk assessment based on high-dose animal exposure experiments. Chem Res Toxicol 5:742–748

Cohen SM, Ellwein LB, Okamura T, et al (1991) Comparative bladder tumor promoting activity of sodium saccharin, sodium ascorbate, related acids, and calcium salts in rats. Cancer Res 51:1766–1777

Cohen SM, Fisher MJ, Sakata T, et al (1990) Comparative analysis of the proliferative response of the rat urinary bladder to sodium saccharin by light and scanning electron microscopy and autoradiography. Scan Microsc 4:135–142

Cohen SM, Murasaki G, Fukushima S, Greenfield RE (1982) Effect of regenerative hyperplasia on the urinary bladder: Carcinogenicity of sodium saccharin and *N*-[4-(5-nitro-2-furyl)-2-thiazolyl]formamide. Cancer Res 42:65–71

Columbano A, Rajalakshmi S, Sarma DSR (1981) Requirement of cell proliferation for the initiation of liver carcinogenesis as assayed by three different procedures. Cancer Res 41:2079–2083

Corley RA (1994) Adaptive metabolic and pathologic changes following chronic inhalation of propylene glycol monomethyl ether in rats and mice. Proceedings of INRS Glycol Ethers Symposium, Nancy, France.

Davies TS, Monro A (1995) Marketed human pharmaceuticals reported to be tumorigenic in rodents. J Am College Toxicol 14:90–107

Doolittle DJ, Muller G, Scribner HE (1987) Relationship between hepatotoxicity and induction of replicative DNA synthesis following single or multiple doses of carbon tetrachloride. J Toxicol Environ Health 22:63–78

Drinkwater NR (1994) Genetic control of hepatocarcinogenesis in C3H mice. Drug Metabol Rev 26:201–208

Ellwein LB, Cohen SM (1988) A cellular dynamics model of experimental bladder cancer: Analysis of sodium saccharin in the rat. Risk Anal 8:215–221

Ellwein LB, Cohen SM (1990) The health risks of saccharin revisited. Crit Rev Toxicol 20:311–326

Faccini JM, Butler WR, Friedmann JC, et al. (1992) IFSTP guidelines for the design and interpretation of the chronic rodent carcinogenicity bioassay. Exp Toxicol Pathol 44:443–456

Farber E (1980) The sequential analysis of liver cancer induction. Biochim Biophys Acta 605:149–166

Fausto N, Shank PR (1983) Oncogene expression in liver regeneration and hepatocarcinogenesis. Hepatology 3:1016–1023

Flamm GW, Lehman-McKeeman LD (1991) The human relevance of the renal tumor-inducing potential of d-limonene in male rats: implications for risk assessment. Regulat Toxicol Pharmacol 13:70–86

Frederick CB, Dooley KL, Kodell RL, et al (1989) The effect of lifetime sodium saccharin dosing on mice initiated with the carcinogen 2-acetylaminofluorene. Fund Appl Toxicol 12:346–357

Fry RJM, Storer JB (1987) External radiation carcinogenesis. Adv Radiat Biol 13:31–90

Fukushima S, Cohen SM (1980) Saccharin-induced hyperplasia of the rat urinary bladder. Cancer Res 40:734–736

Garland EM, Shapiro R, Kraft PL, et al (1991) Effects of *in utero* and postnatal sodium saccharin exposure on the nutritional status of the young rat. II. Dose response and reversibility. Food Chem Toxicol 29:669–679

Gehring PJ, Watanabe PG, Park CN (1978) Resolution of dose-response toxicity data for chemicals requiring metabolic activation. Example—vinyl chloride. Toxicol Appl Pharmacol 44:581–591

Gehring PJ, Watanabe PG, Young JD (1977) The relevance of dose-dependent pharmacokinetics in the assessment of carcinogenic hazard of chemicals. In ???? (eds), Origins of Human Cancer. Cold Spring Harbor Laboratory, Cold Spring Harbor, NY, pp 187–203

Goldsworthy TL, Hanigan MH, Pitot HC (1986) Models of hepatocarcinogenesis in the rat—contrasts and comparisons. Crit Rev Toxicol 17:61–89

Goldsworthy TL, Lyght O, Burnett VL, Popp JA (1987) Potential role of $\alpha 2\mu$-globulin protein droplet accumulation and cell replication in the renal carcinogenicity of rats exposed to trichloroethylene, perchloroethylene and pentachloroethane. Tox Appl Pharmacol 96:367–379

Hasegawa R, Greenfield RE, Murasaki G, et al (1985) Initiation of urinary bladder carcinogenesis in rats by freeze ulceration with sodium saccharin promotion. Cancer Res 45:1469–1473

Haseman JK, Lockhart A (1994) The relationship between use of the maximum tolerated dose and study sensitivity for detecting rodent carcinogenicity. Fund Appl Toxicol 22:82–91

Heck Hd'A (1987) Bladder stones and bladder cancer: a review of the toxicology of terephthalic acid. In Butterworth BE, Slaga TJ (eds), Nongenotoxic Mechanisms in Carcinogenesis. Banbury Report 25. Cold Spring Harbor Laboratory, Cold Spring Harbor, NY, pp 233–243

Hiraga K, Fujii T (1981) Induction of tumors of the urinary system in F344 rats by dietary administration of sodium o-phenylphenate. Food Cosmet Toxicol 19:303–310

Hoel DG, Kaplan NL, Anderson MW (1983) Implications of nonlinear kinetics on risk estimation in carcinogenesis. Science 219:1032–1037

International Agency for Research on Cancer (1980) Monographs on the Evaluation of Carcinogenic Risk of Chemicals to Humans, Vol. 22. International Agency for Research on Cancer, Lyons, France, pp 111–170

International Programme on Chemical Safety (1994) Chloroform. Environmental Health Criteria 163. World Health Organization, Geneva.

Jorgenson TA, Meierhenry EF, Rushbrook CJ, et al (1985) Carcinogenicity of chloroform in drinking water to male Osborne–Mendel rats and female B6C3F$_1$ mice. Fundam Appl Toxicol 5:760–769

Kubic VL, Anders MW, Engel RR, et al. (1974) Metabolism of dihalomethanes to carbon dioxide. I. Drug Metab Dispos 2:53–57

Landry TD, Gushow TS, Yano BL (1983) Propylene glycol monomethyl ether: A 13-week inhalation toxicity study in rats and rabbits. Fund Appl Toxicol 3:627–630

Larson JL, Templin MV, Wolf DC, et al (1996) A 90-day chloroform inhalation study in female and male B6C3F1 mice: Implications for cancer risk assessment. Fundam Appl Toxicol 30:118–137

Larson JL, Wolf DC, Butterworth BE (1994) Induced cytotoxicity and cell proliferation in the hepatocarcinogenicity of chloroform in female B6C3F$_1$ mice: Comparison of administration by gavage in corn oil vs. ad libitum in drinking water. Fundam Appl Toxicol 22:90–102

Larson JL, Wolf DC, Butterworth BE (1995) Induced regenerative cell proliferation in livers and kidneys of male F-344 rats given chloroform in corn oil by gavage or ad libitum in drinking water. Toxicology 95:73–86

Lefevre PA, Tinwell H, Galloway SM, et al. (1994) Evaluation of the genetic toxicity of the peroxisome proliferator and carcinogen methyl clofenipate. Human Exp Toxicol, in press.

Loeb LA (1991) Mutator phenotype may be required for multistage carcinogenesis. Cancer Res 51:3075–3079

Loury DJ, Goldsworthy TL, Butterworth BE (1987) The value of measuring cell replication as a predictive index of tissue-specific tumorigenic potential. In Butterworth BE, Slaga TJ (eds), Nongenotoxic Mechanisms in Carcinogenesis. Banbury Report 25. Cold Spring Harbor Laboratory, Cold Spring Harbor, NY, pp 119–136

Maltoni C, Lefemine G (1975) Carcinogenic bioassays of vinyl chloride: current results. Ann NY Acad Sci 246:195–224

Marsman DS, Popp JA (1989) Importance of basophilic hepatocellular foci in the development of hepatic tumors induced by the peroxisome proliferator

Wy-14,643. Proc Am Assoc Cancer Res 30:193.

Mead JE, Fausto N (1989) Transforming growth factor alpha may be a physiological regulator of liver regeneration by means of an autocrine mechanism. Proc Natl Acad Sci 86:1558–1562

Miller JA, Miller EC (1977) Ultimate carcinogens as reactive mutagenic electrophiles. In Hiatt HH, Watson JD, Winstein JA (eds), Origins of Human Cancer. Cold Spring Harbor Laboratory, Cold Spring Harbor, NY, pp 605–628

Miller RR, Hermann EA, Langvardt PW, et al (1983) Comparative metabolism and disposition of ethylene glycol monomethyl ether (EGME) and propylene glycol monomethyl ether (PGME) in male rats. Toxicol Appl Pharmacol 67:229–237

Mirsalis J, Monforte JA, Winegar RA (1994) Transgenic animal models for measuring mutations *in vivo*. Crit Rev Toxicol 24:255–280

Mitchell JR, Jollow DJ, Potter WZ, et al. (1973) Acetaminophen induced hepatic necrosis. J Pharmacol Exp Ther 187:211–217

Morgott DA, Nolan RJ (1987) Nonlinear kinetics of inhaled propylene glycol monomethyl ether in Fischer 344 rats following single and repeated exposures. Toxicol Appl Pharmacol 89:19–28

Morrison V, Ashby J (1994) Reconciliation of five negative and four positive reports of the activity of dimethylnitrosamine in the mouse bone marrow micronucleus assay. Mutagenesis 9:361–365

Murasaki G, Cohen SM (1981) Effect of dose of sodium saccharin on the induction of rat urinary-bladder proliferation. Cancer Res 41:942–944

Nakanishi K, Hagiwara A, Shibata M, et al (1980) Dose-response of saccharin in induction of urinary bladder hyperplasia in Fischer 344 rats pretreated with *N*-butyl-*N*-(4-hydroxybutyl)nitrosamine. J Natl Cancer Inst 65:1005–1010

National Cancer Institute (1976) Carcinogenesis Bioassay of Chloroform. National Technical Information Service No. PB264018/AS. National Cancer Institute, Bethesda, MD

National Toxicology Program (1985) NTP technical report on the toxicology and carcinogenesis studies of dichloromethane in F344/N rats and B6C3F1 mice (inhalation studies). NTP-TR-306.

Perera FP (1991) Perspectives on the risk assessment for non-genotoxic carcinogens and tumour promoters. Environ Health Perspect 94:231–235

Rao KS, Watanabe PG, Gehring PJ (1985) Toxicologic data in chemical safety evaluation. In ???? (eds), Patty's Industrial Hygiene and Toxicology, Vol. 3b, 2nd ed. Wiley, New York, pp 27–74

Reitz RH, Fox TR, Quast JF, et al (1983) Molecular mechanisms involved in the toxicity of orthophenyphenol and its sodium salt. Chem-Biol Interact 43:99–119

Reitz RH, Fox TR, Quast JF, et al (1984) Biochemical factors involved in the effects of orthophenylphenol (OPP) and sodium orthophenylphenol (SOPP) on the urinary tract of male F344 rats. Toxicol Appl Pharmacol 73:345–349

Reitz RH, Mendrala AL, Corley RA, et al (1990) Estimating the risk of liver cancer associated with human exposures to chloroform. Toxicol Appl Pharmacol 105:443–459

Reitz RH, Mendrala AL, Guengerich FP (1989) In vitro metabolism of methylene chloride in human and animal tissues: use of physiologically-based pharmacokinetic models. Toxicol Appl Pharmacol 97:230–246

Reitz RH, Mendrala AL, Park CN (1988) Incorporation of in vitro enzyme data into the physiologically based pharmacokinetic (PB-PK) model for methylene chloride: implication for risk assessment. Toxicol Lett 43:97–116

Richardson FC, Boucheron JA, Dyroff M, et al (1986) Biochemical and morphological studies of heterogeneous lobe responses in hepatocarcinogenesis. Carcinogenesis 7:247–251

Schoenig GP, Goldenthal EI, Geil RG, et al (1985) Evaluation of the dose response and *in utero* exposure to saccharin in the rat. Food Chem Toxicol 23:475–490

Schroter C, Parzefall W, Schroter H, Schulte-Hermann R (1987) Dose-response studies on the effects of *a*-, *b*-, and *g*-hexachlorocyclohexane on putative preneoplastic foci, monooxygenases, and growth in rat liver. Cancer Res 47:80–88

Schulte-Hermann R, Ochs H, Bursch W, Parzefall W (1988) Quantitative structure-activity studies on effects of sixteen different steroids on growth and monooxygenases of rat liver. Cancer Res 48:2462–2468

Schulte-Hermann R, Schuppler J, Timmermann-Trosiener I, et al (1983) The role of growth of normal and preneoplastic cell populations for tumor promotion in rat liver. Environ Health Perspect 50:185–194

Serota D, Ulland B, Carlborg F (1984) Hazleton chronic oral study in mice: Methylene Chloride. Food Solvents Workshop I. Bethesda, MD

Shelby MD, Erexson GL, Hook GJ, Tice RR (1993) Evaluation of a three exposure mouse bone marrow micronucleus protocol: results with 49 chemicals. Environ Mol Mutagen 21:160–179

Starr TB (1989) Quantitative cancer risk estimation for formaldehyde. In Feron VJ, Bosland MC (eds), Nasal Carcinogenesis in Rodents. Wageningen, Pudaoc, The Netherlands, pp 179–184

Stott WT, Reitz RH, Schumann AM, Watanabe PG (1981) Genetic and nongenetic events in neoplasia. Food Cosmet Toxicol 19:567–576

Swenberg JA (1993) $\alpha 2\mu$-globulin nephropathy: review of the cellular and molecular mechanisms involved and their implications for human risk assessment. Environ Health Perspect 101(Suppl 6):39–44

Swenberg JA, Maronpot RR (1991) Chemically induced cell proliferation as a criterion in selecting doses for long-term bioassays. In Butterworth BE, Slaga TJ, McClain M (eds), Chemically Induced Cell Proliferation: Implications for Risk Assessment. Wiley-Liss, New York, pp 245–251

Templin MV, Jamison KC, Wolf DC, et al (1995) Comparison of chloroform-induced toxicity in the kidneys, liver, and nasal passages of male Osborne-Mendel and F344 rats. Cancer Letters, in press.

Templin MV, Jamison KC, Wolf DC, Butterworth BE (1996a) Chloroform-induced cytotoxicity in BDF_1 mice. The Toxicologist 30:134

Templin MV, Larson JL, Butterworth BE, et al (1996b) A 90-day chloroform inhalation study in male and female F-344 rats: Profile of toxicity and relevance to bioassay results. Fundam Appl Toxicol, in press

Tennant RW, Margolin BW, Shelby MD, et al. (1987) Prediction of chemical carcinogenicity in rodents from *in vitro* genetic toxicity assays. Science 236:933–941

Tinwell H, Ashby J (1994) Comparative activity of human carcinogens and NTP rodent carcinogens in the mouse bone-marrow micronucleus assay: an integrative approach to genetic toxicity data assessment. Env Health Perspect 102:758–762

US Environmental Protection Agency (1991) α_{2u}-globulin: Association with chemically induced renal toxicity and neoplasia in the male rat. EPA/625/3-91/019F. Risk Assessment Forum, US Environmental Protection Agency, Washington, DC

Vogel EW (1989) Nucleophilic selectivity of carcinogens as a determinant of enhanced mutational response. Carcinogenesis 10:2093–2106

Walker VE, Fennell TR, Boucheron JA, et al (1990) Macromolecular adducts of ethylene oxide: a literature review and a time-course study on the formation of 7-(2-hydroxyethyl)guanine following exposures of rats by inhalation. Mutat Res 233:151–164

West RW, Sheldon WG, Gaylor DW, et al (1986) The effects of saccharin on the development of neoplastic lesions initiated with *N*-Methyl-*N*-nitrosourea in the rat urothelium. Fund Appl Toxicol 7:585–600

Yamamoto S, Aiso S, Ikawa N, Matsushima T (1994) Japan Bioassay Laboratory, Japan Industrial Safety and Health Association, 2445

Ohshibahara Hirasawa Hando Kanagawa, 257 Japan. Carcinogenesis studies of chloroform in F344 rats and BDF_1 mice (abstract). Proceedings of the Fifty-third Annual Meeting of the Japanese Cancer Association.